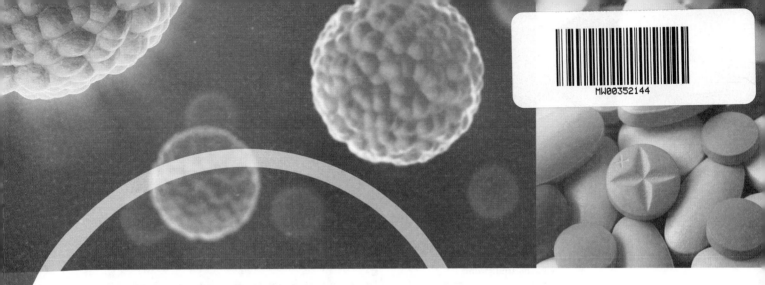

STUDY GUIDE FOR
PHARMACOLOGY FOR
HEALTH PROFESSIONALS

SECOND EDITION

W. Renée Acosta, RPh, MS
College of Pharmacy
University of Texas at Austin

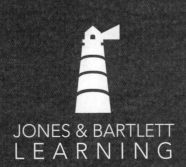

JONES & BARTLETT
LEARNING

World Headquarters
Jones & Bartlett Learning
5 Wall Street
Burlington, MA 01803
978-443-5000
info@jblearning.com
www.jblearning.com

Jones & Bartlett Learning books and products are available through most bookstores and online book-sellers. To contact Jones & Bartlett Learning directly, call 800-832-0034, fax 978-443-8000, or visit our website, www.jblearning.com.

Substantial discounts on bulk quantities of Jones & Bartlett Learning publications are available to corporations, professional associations, and other qualified organizations. For details and specific discount information, contact the special sales department at Jones & Bartlett Learning via the above contact information or send an email to special-sales@jblearning.com.

29447-7

Production Credits

VP, Product Management: Amanda Martin
Director of Product Management: Cathy L. Esperti
Product Specialist: Ashley Malone
Product Coordinator: Elena Sorrentino
Digital Project Specialist: Angela Dooley
Director of Marketing: Andrea DeFronzo
Marketing Manager: Suzy Balk
Production Services Manager: Colleen Lamy
VP, Manufacturing and Inventory Control: Therese Connell
Product Fulfillment Manager: Wendy Kilborn
Composition: S4Carlisle Publishing Services
Project Management: S4Carlisle Publishing Services
Cover & Text Design: Briana Yates
Senior Media Development Editor: Faith Brosnan
Rights Specialist: Becky Damon
Cover Image (Title Page, Part Opener, Chapter Opener): © Henrik5000/Shutterstock
© FotografiaBasica/Getty Images
Printing and Binding: McNaughton & Gunn

Library of Congress Cataloging-in-Publication Data
Library of Congress Cataloging-in-Publication Data unavailable at time of printing.

LCCN: 2020935614

6048

Printed in the United States of America
24 23 22 21 20   10 9 8 7 6 5 4 3 2 1

INTRODUCTION

Study Guide for Pharmacology for Health Professionals, second edition, is a companion to the textbook, *Pharmacology for Health Professionals*, second edition, by W. Renée Acosta. The study guide is designed for use in conjunction with the companion textbook or other texts to be used in undergraduate pharmacology courses for health professions students.

The study guide reinforces the concepts of the main text with a variety of question types, including:

- Matching
- Multiple Choice
- True/False
- Recall Facts
- Fill in the Blanks
- List
- Clinical Applications
- Case Studies

The 46 chapters match the contents of *Pharmacology for Health Professionals*, second edition. The questions cover a broad range of information learned in a typical undergraduate pharmacology course. A complete Answer Key is available for instructors. To learn more, please contact your Jones & Bartlett Learning Account Representative.

CONTENTS

1

General Principles of Pharmacology

I. MATCH THE FOLLOWING

Match the term from Column A with the correct definition from Column B.

COLUMN A

____ 1. Additive drug reaction
____ 2. Antagonist
____ 3. Agonist
____ 4. Controlled substance
____ 5. Hypersensitivity
____ 6. Pharmaceutic phase
____ 7. Pharmacokinetics
____ 8. Polypharmacy
____ 9. Receptor
____ 10. Teratogen

COLUMN B

A. Taking of numerous drugs that can potentially react with one another

B. Any substance that causes abnormal development of the fetus

C. Drugs with a high potential for abuse that are controlled by special regulations

D. A specialized macromolecule that binds to the drug molecule, altering the function of the cell and producing the therapeutic response

E. Activities occurring within the body after a drug is administered

F. Being allergic to a drug

G. A drug that binds with a receptor to produce a therapeutic response

H. A drug that joins with a receptor to prevent the action of an agonist at that receptor

I. A reaction that occurs when the combined effect of two drugs is equal to the sum of each drug given alone

J. The dissolution of the drug

II. MATCH THE FOLLOWING

Match the item from Column A with the correct definition from Column B.

COLUMN A

_____ 1. Pure food and drug act 1906

_____ 2. Harrison narcotic act 1914

_____ 3. Pure food, drug, and cosmetic act 1938

_____ 4. Controlled substance act 1970

_____ 5. Comprehensive drug abuse prevention and control act 1970

_____ 6. Drug enforcement agency (DEA)

_____ 7. Food and drug administration (FDA)

_____ 8. Dietary supplement health and education act (DSHEA)

_____ 9. Orphan drug act 1983

_____ 10. Investigational new drug (IND)

COLUMN B

A. Chief federal agency responsible for enforcing the Controlled Substances Act

B. Agency responsible for approving new drugs and monitoring drugs for adverse or toxic reactions

C. Law that gives the FDA control over the manufacture and sale of drugs, food, and cosmetics

D. First law that regulated the sale of narcotic drugs

E. Regulates the manufacture, distribution, and dispensation of drugs with a potential for abuse

F. First attempt by the U.S. government to regulate and control the manufacture, distribution, and sale of drugs

G. Title II of the Comprehensive Drug Abuse Prevention and Control Act that deals with the control and enforcement of the Act

H. Act that defines herbs, vitamins, minerals, amino acids, and other natural supplements and permits general health claims as long as a disclaimer is present

I. Encourages the development and marketing of products used to treat rare diseases

J. The clinical testing phase of drug approval by the FDA

III. TRUE OR FALSE

Indicate whether each statement is True (T) or False (F).

_____ 1. A New Drug Application (NDA) is submitted immediately following Phase II of the clinical testing portion of the IND status.

_____ 2. The accelerated approval of drugs by the FDA seeks to make lifesaving investigational drugs available for health care providers to administer in early Phase I and II clinical trials.

_____ 3. The compassionate access program allows drugs to be given free of charge to patients in financial need.

_____ 4. Legend drugs can be prescribed by any health care provider.

_____ 5. Prescriptions for controlled substances must be written in ink and must include the name and address of the patient and the DEA number of the health care provider.

_____ 6. All drugs taken by mouth, except liquids, go through three phases: the pharmaceutic phase, the pharmacokinetic phase, and the pharmacodynamic phase.

_____ 7. The absorption of a drug is the process that refers to the metabolic activities involving the drug within the body after it is administered.

_____ 8. All drugs produce more than one effect on the body.

_____ 9. An allergic reaction to a drug occurs because the patient's immune system views the drug as an antibody.

_____ 10. Drug toxicity can be reversible or irreversible.

_____ 11. A pharmacogenetic disorder is a genetically caused abnormal response to a normal dose of a drug.

IV. MULTIPLE CHOICE

Circle the letter of the best answer.

1. The pre-FDA phase of drug development includes _____.
   a. in vitro testing
   b. development of a drug that looks promising
   c. testing using animal and human cells
   d. testing using live animals
   e. All of the above

2 and 3. The FDA phase of drug development requires the manufacturer of the drug to apply first for (2) _____ and then, after three phases of clinical testing, to apply for a (3) _____.
   a. clinical trial phase I
   b. IND
   c. NDA
   d. clinical trial phase II
   e. clinical trial phase III

4. The MedWatch system allows health care professionals to _____.
   a. track drug use by patients
   b. obtain pharmacy records of patients
   c. monitor prescriptions written by a physician
   d. report observations of serious adverse drug reactions
   e. contact government officials about insurance fraud

5. The Orphan Drug Program allows manufacturers to produce drugs that treat rare disorders; in exchange, the manufacturer may receive _____.
   a. grants
   b. tax incentives
   c. protocol assistance by the FDA
   d. 7 years of exclusive production rights for the drug involved
   e. All of the above

6. A _____ is a drug that the FDA has designated to be potentially harmful unless its use is supervised by a licensed health care provider.
   a. controlled substance
   b. prescription drug
   c. nonprescription drug
   d. legend drug
   e. Both b and d

7. The Drug Enforcement Agency (DEA) _____.
   a. is under the U.S. Department of Justice
   b. enforces the Controlled Substances Act of 1970
   c. requires compliance by all health care workers
   d. can punish those who fail to comply by imprisonment
   e. All of the above

8. Pregnancy Category D drugs, whether prescription or nonprescription, _____.
   a. have a risk that cannot be ruled out
   b. have controlled studies that show no risk
   c. have positive evidence of risk to the human fetus
   d. should never be used during pregnancy
   e. None of the above

9. Pharmacokinetics refers to _____.
   a. absorption
   b. excretion
   c. distribution
   d. metabolism
   e. All of the above

10. The therapeutic level of a drug is the level at which _____.
    a. toxic symptoms may develop
    b. the drug is pharmacologically inactive
    c. the drug is effective
    d. the liver biotransforms the drug
    e. occurs directly after administration

11. Drugs that have some receptor fit and produce a response but inhibit other responses are_____.
    a. agonists
    b. partial agonists
    c. antagonists
    d. partial antagonists
    e. antigens

12. The number of receptor sites available at a target site can _____.
    a. influence the effects of a drug
    b. change as a person ages
    c. allow more potent drugs to be used
    d. keep other drugs from acting
    e. be chemically altered

13. Allergic or hypersensitivity reactions _____.
    a. usually begin to occur after more than one dose of a drug
    b. occur because the patient's immune system views the drug as a foreign substance
    c. must be reported to the health care provider
    d. may occur within minutes after the drug is given
    e. All of the above

14. When a patient develops a tolerance to a drug, _____.
    a. he or she has a decreased response to the drug
    b. he or she requires an increase in dosage to achieve the desired effect
    c. it is an indicator of drug dependence
    d. the patient's body does not metabolize and excrete the drug before the next dose is given
    e. Answers a, b, and c

15. Drug interactions may occur _____.
    a. between two drugs
    b. between oral drugs and food
    c. between a drug and alcohol
    d. All of the above
    e. a and b only

16. A patient's response to a drug may be influenced by which of the following factors?
    a. Disease
    b. Age
    c. Weight
    d. Gender
    e. All of the above

17. Drug response can be greatly affected by:
    a. liver disease
    b. kidney disease
    c. elderly patient
    d. very young patient
    e. All of the above

18. The route of administration of a drug may influence a patient's drug response. The route order of response from most rapid to least rapid is _____.
    a. IV, IM, subcutaneous, and oral
    b. IM, subcutaneous, oral, and IV
    c. subcutaneous, oral, IV, and IM
    d. oral, IM, subcutaneous, and IV
    e. None of the above

V. RECALL FACTS

Indicate which of the following statements are facts with an F. If the statement is not a fact, leave the line blank.

ABOUT TOXIC REACTIONS/LEVELS

____ 1. Can occur when drugs are administered in large doses

____ 2. Some reactions are immediate while others may not be seen for months

____ 3. Can be reversible or irreversible

____ 4. Patients always know when a toxic reaction is going to occur

____ 5. Can occur in recommended doses

____ 6. Only licensed health care providers need to know the signs and symptoms of toxicity

ABOUT CONTROLLED SUBSTANCES

____ 1. Have a high potential for abuse

____ 2. May cause physical or psychological dependence

____ 3. Prescriptions for these drugs cannot be filled more than 6 months after the prescription was written

____ 4. Prescriptions for these drugs cannot be refilled more than five times

____ 5. Are the largest category of drugs

____ 6. Are categorized in five schedules, C-I through C-V

ABOUT DRUG HALF-LIFE

____ 1. 98% of drugs are eliminated in five to six half-lives

____ 2. Increases with liver or kidney disease

____ 3. Is the same for the same drug in most people

____ 4. Can be altered by changing the dose

____ 5. Is based on the frequency of administration

____ 6. Is the time required for the body to eliminate 50% of the drug

VI. FILL IN THE BLANKS

Fill in the blanks using words from the list below.

cellular	small	2–10	G6PD	psychological	pharmacokinetics
8–12	physical	immediate	generic		

1. The three phases of clinical testing of a new drug can last anywhere from _____ years.

2. _____ dependency is a compulsive need to use a substance repeatedly to avoid mild to severe withdrawal symptoms.

3. _____ dependency is a compulsion to use a substance to obtain a pleasurable experience.

4. In hospitals or other agencies that dispense controlled substances, scheduled drugs are counted every _____ hours.

5. Enteric coated drugs do not disintegrate until they reach the _____ intestine.

6. Most drugs act on the body by altering _____ function.

7. Changes that occur with aging affect the _____ of a drug.

8. Individuals with _____ deficiency have abnormal reactions to a number of drugs.

9. Anaphylactic shock is a serious allergic drug reaction that requires _____ medical attention.

10. The _____ name of a drug is defined as the name given to a drug before it becomes official and may be used in all countries, by all manufacturers, and is not capitalized.

VII. LIST

List the requested number of items.

1. List the three categories to which the FDA assigns a new drug.

   a. _____

   b. _____

   c. _____

2. List four items that *must* be on a prescription for a drug.

   a. _____

   b. _____

   c. _____

   d. _____

3. List four items that *must* be on the product label of an OTC drug.

   a. _____

   b. _____

   c. _____

   d. _____

4. List the two phases that liquid and parenteral drugs go through in the body.

   a. _____

   b. _____

5. List the four activities that pharmacokinetics involves.

   a. _____

   b. _____

   c. _____

   d. _____

6. List the seven types of drug reactions in the body.

   a. _____

   b. _____

   c. _____

   d. _____

   e. _____

   f. _____

   g. _____

7. List the three effects of drug–drug interactions.

   a. _____

   b. _____

   c. _____

8. List the five schedules of controlled substances and give a brief definition.

   a. _____

   b. _____

   c. _____

   d. _____

   e. _____

9. List the four names that a drug may have.

   a. _____

   b. _____

   c. _____

   d. _____

10. List the five Pregnancy Categories and give a brief definition.

   a. _____

   b. _____

   c. _____

   d. _____

   e. _____

VIII. CLINICAL APPLICATIONS

1. Your overweight neighbor, knowing that you are in health care, wants to know why her prescription for antibiotics is the same strength as her elderly father who has kidney disease, but the other medication that they both take for cholesterol control has different dosages and schedules. What might you tell your neighbor in response?

IX. CASE STUDY

Mr. Jones has a disease for which there is no current FDA approved treatment. His physician, Dr. Goldstein, has told him that there is a drug in clinical trials that has shown a great deal of promise in treating his condition. Dr. Goldstein contacts the company that is conducting the trial and receives permission to use the drug with Mr. Jones.

1. This is an example of

   a. the Orphan Drug Program.
   b. accelerated approval.
   c. compassionate access to unapproved drugs.
   d. DEA enforcement.

2. Mr. Jones is very sick. His disease has caused his kidneys to not function as well. He is at increased risk for:

   a. pharmacogenetic reactions.
   b. drug–drug interactions.
   c. drug–food interactions.
   d. toxic reactions.

3. The role of the pharmaceutical company is to

   a. analyze and present to the FDA data about this treatment.
   b. provide the drug free to the patient.
   c. make a proposal to the FDA to target patients with the disease.
   d. All of the above

2

The Administration of Drugs

I. MATCH THE FOLLOWING

Match the term from Column A with the correct definition from Column B.

COLUMN A

____ 1. Extravasation
____ 2. Inhalation
____ 3. Intradermal
____ 4. Intramuscular
____ 5. Intravenous
____ 6. Parenteral
____ 7. Subcutaneous
____ 8. Sublingual
____ 9. Transdermal
____ 10. Unit dose

COLUMN B

A. The escape of fluid from a blood vessel into the surrounding tissues

B. Route of administration in which the drug is injected into the muscle tissue

C. Route of administration in which the drug is injected into the skin tissue

D. Route of administration in which the drug is injected just below the layer of skin

E. Route of administration in which the drug is absorbed through the skin from a patch

F. Route of administration in which drug droplets, vapor, or gas is inhaled and absorbed through the mucous membranes of the respiratory tract

G. Route of administration in which the drug is injected into a vein

H. A single dose of a drug packaged ready for patient use

I. Route of administration in which the drug is placed under the tongue for absorption

J. A general term for drug administration in which the drug is injected inside the body

II. TRUE OR FALSE

Indicate whether each statement is True (T) or False (F).

____ 1. A drug error is any occurrence that can cause a patient to receive the wrong dose, the wrong drug, the wrong route, or the drug at the wrong time.

____ 2. A STAT order is an order to administer a drug as needed.

____ 3. A standing order is an order written when a patient is to receive the prescribed drug on a regular basis.

____ 4. An advantage of once-a-week dosing is that the patient who experiences mild adverse reactions would only have to experience them once in a week rather than every day.

____ 5. New OSHA guidelines help to reduce needle-stick injuries among health care workers and others who handle medical sharps.

____ 6. Many needlestick injuries can be prevented with the use of safe needle devices.

____ 7. A subcutaneous injection places the drug into tissues below the muscle level.

____ 8. The Z-track method of IM injection is used when a drug is highly irritating to subcutaneous tissues or may permanently stain the skin.

_____ 9. Whenever a drug is added to an IV fluid, the IV bag must have an attached label indicating the drug and the dose added.

_____ 10. After an IV infusion is started, if either extravasation or infiltration occurs the infusion must be stopped and restarted in another vein.

_____ 11. Drugs administered by the transdermal route are readily absorbed through the skin and have systemic effects.

_____ 12. Topical drugs act on the skin but are not absorbed through the skin.

III. MULTIPLE CHOICE

Circle the letter of the best answer.

1. When a drug error occurs, the health care worker should _____.
   a. wait to see if any adverse effects occur
   b. report the incident immediately
   c. not tell anyone so they do not get into trouble
   d. tell the patient not to worry
   e. None of the above

2. In a computerized dispensing system the _____.
   a. drug orders are filled and medications are dispensed to fill each patient's medication order for a 24-hour period
   b. drugs that are dispensed are automatically recorded in a computerized system
   c. bar code scanner is used to record and charge routine and PRN drugs
   d. drugs most frequently ordered are kept on the unit in containers in a designated medication room
   e. All of the above

3. Health care professionals who are involved in drug administration should know _____.
   a. the reason why the drug is used
   b. the drug's general actions and adverse reactions
   c. special precautions in administration
   d. normal dose ranges
   e. All of the above

4. Oral route drug administration _____.
   a. is the most frequent route of administration
   b. rarely causes physical discomfort
   c. is relatively easy for patients who are alert and can swallow
   d. can use drug forms such as tablets, capsules, or liquids
   e. All of the above

5. A method of parenteral drug administration is _____.
   a. subcutaneous
   b. intramuscular
   c. intravenous
   d. intradermal
   e. All of the above

6. Parenteral routes of administration that require special devices and materials can include _____.
   a. intra-articular
   b. intra-arterial
   c. intracardiac
   d. All of the above

7. Drugs administered by the subcutaneous route _____.
   a. are absorbed more slowly than intramuscular drugs
   b. are delivered into the tissues between the skin and the muscle
   c. can be given in large amounts (>1 ml)
   d. are generally given in the upper arm, upper back, or upper abdomen
   e. Answers a, b, and d

8. Sites for the administration of intramuscular drugs are _____.
   a. deltoid muscle
   b. ventrogluteal muscle
   c. dorsogluteal muscle
   d. vastus lateralis muscle
   e. All of the above

9. Infusion controllers and infusion pumps are electronic infusion devices. The primary difference between the two is that _____.
   a. an infusion pump administers the infused drug under pressure, and an infusion controller does not add pressure
   b. an infusion pump administers the infused drug without added pressure, whereas an infusion controller adds pressure
   c. both devices administer the drug under pressure; the difference is the amount of pressure used
   d. there is no difference; the two devices are the same
   e. None of the above

10. Intradermal drug administration _____.
   a. usually results in the formation of a wheal
   b. requires a 90 degree angle of needle insertion
   c. provides good results for allergy testing or local anesthesia
   d. requires a portal to be implanted in the skin
   e. Both a and c

IV. RECALL FACTS

Indicate which of the following statements are facts with an F. If the statement is not a fact, leave the line blank.

ABOUT IV DRUG ADMINISTRATION

_____ 1. Are given directly into the blood by a needle inserted into a vein

_____ 2. Drug action occurs almost immediately

_____ 3. May be given slowly (>1 minute) or rapidly (IV Push)

_____ 4. Can be delivered by an IV port or through a heparin lock

ABOUT TRANSDERMAL DRUG ADMINISTRATION

_____ 1. Allows the drug to be readily absorbed from the skin and have systemic effects

_____ 2. Allows for a relatively constant blood concentration

_____ 3. Increases the risk of toxicity

_____ 4. The sites are rotated to prevent skin irritation

_____ 5. Should have the site shaved of hair before administration

_____ 6. Old patches are removed when a new dose is applied

ABOUT AFTER A DRUG IS ADMINISTERED

_____ 1. Is always documented as soon as possible

_____ 2. The patient's response to the drug is monitored.

_____ 3. The patient's vital signs are not taken until several hours after the drug is administered.

_____ 4. IV flow rate, site used, or problems with administration are recorded

_____ 5. Adverse reactions are recorded at 15-minute intervals

ABOUT WRITTEN DRUG ORDERS

_____ 1. Should include the patient's name

_____ 2. Should include the name of the drug to be administered

_____ 3. Should include who is to administer the drug

_____ 4. Should include what dosage, route, and form of the drug are to be used

_____ 5. Should be written by the prescriber except in an emergency situation.

_____ 6. Should include the frequency of administration

ABOUT GUIDELINES FOR PREPARING A DRUG FOR ADMINISTRATION

_____ 1. The written orders should be checked

_____ 2. The drug label should be checked only once

_____ 3. Never remove a drug from an unlabeled container

_____ 4. Deposit capsules and tablets into clean hands then drop into medicine cup

_____ 5. Replace the caps of drug containers immediately after the drug is removed.

_____ 6. Return drugs requiring special storage immediately to their storage area.

_____ 7. Follow aseptic technique when handling syringes and needles.

ABOUT PATIENT CARE CONSIDERATIONS FOR ORAL DRUG ADMINISTRATION

_____ 1. A full glass of water should be available to the patient

_____ 2. The patient may take the oral drug in any position.

_____ 3. The health care provider may safely leave the drug for the patient to take when convenient.

_____ 4. Patients with nasogastric feeding tubes may have their medication given through the tube.

_____ 5. Sublingual drugs must not be chewed or swallowed.

ABOUT PATIENT CARE CONSIDERATIONS FOR PARENTERAL DRUG ADMINISTRATION

_____ 1. Gloves must be worn for protection from a potential blood spill.

_____ 2. Cleanse the skin at the site of injection.

_____ 3. After insertion of the needle for an IM injection, blood should appear in the syringe after pulling back on the barrel.

_____ 4. Syringes are not recapped but are disposed of according to policy.

_____ 5. There is no need to place pressure on an injection site from an IV, subcutaneous, or IM injection.

V. FILL IN THE BLANKS

Fill in the blanks using words from the list below

11	circular	standing	outward	skin	inner
muscle	administration	topical	inhalation	immediately	

1. When a drug error occurs it must be reported
   _____.

2. Many drug errors are made during
   _____.

3. A _____ order is one that is written when the patient is to receive the prescribed drug on a regular basis.

4. The skin site for parenteral drug administration is cleansed using a(n) _____ motion from a(n) _____ point and moving _____.

5. A Sharps Injury Log must be kept by employers with _____ or more employees.

6. A subcutaneous injection places the drug into the tissues between the _____ and the _____.

7. Drugs that are used to soften, disinfect, or lubricate the skin are _____ drugs.

8. Examples of drugs administered by _____ include mucolytics, anti-inflammatories, and bronchodilators.

VI. LIST

List the requested number of items.

1. List the six rights of drug administration.
   a. _____
   b. _____
   c. _____
   d. _____
   e. _____
   f. _____

2. List the three times that a drug label should be checked.
   a. _____
   b. _____
   c. _____

3. List the three forms of oral drugs.
   a. _____
   b. _____
   c. _____

4. List the four most commonly used routes of administration of parenteral drugs.
   a. _____
   b. _____
   c. _____
   d. _____

5. List six diseases that can be transmitted by needle exposures or sticks.
   a. _____
   b. _____
   c. _____
   d. _____
   e. _____
   f. _____

6. List three sites for subcutaneous injections.
   a. _____
   b. _____
   c. _____

7. List six ways that a drug may be administered via the IV route:

   a. _____

   b. _____

   c. _____

   d. _____

   e. _____

   f. _____

8. List five items that should be on a written drug order.

   a. _____

   b. _____

   c. _____

   d. _____

   e. _____

9. List ten forms of topical and mucous membrane applications.

   a. _____

   b. _____

   c. _____

   d. _____

   e. _____

   f. _____

   g. _____

   h. _____

   i. _____

   j. _____

VII. CLINICAL APPLICATIONS

1. Mr. T is being discharged from the hospital but will need to continue his medications at home. As a health care professional, what might you ask or suggest to Mr. T regarding his home environment and safe drug administration?

2. Today is the first day of employment for Miss C in a clinical setting of more than 20 persons. What OSHA guidelines should she be informed of before she begins using needles?

VIII. CASE STUDY

Sue Jones has just received an intravenous medication to terminate an abnormal heart rhythm she was having. The medication was given through a heparin lock. Patency of the heparin lock/IV is a major concern during intravenous medication administration. After the injection, the health professional, Mr. Smith, notices that there is swelling at the needle site.

1. This probably means that the site is
   a. infiltrated.
   b. infected.
   c. patent.
   d. inflamed.

2. What should Mr. Smith do?
   a. Administer more fluid through the heparin lock
   b. Administer another dose of medication through the heparin lock
   c. Insert a new IV catheter and remove the old one
   d. Nothing

3. Mr. Smith is concerned that the medication leakage may have a damaging effect on the tissue at the old IV site. This escape of fluid from the blood vessel into the surrounding tissue is called
   a. infiltration.
   b. extravasation.
   c. inhalation.
   d. Z-track.

3

Math Review

I. MATCH THE FOLLOWING

Match the term from Column A with the correct definition from Column B.

COLUMN A

_____ 1. Common fraction
_____ 2. Denominator
_____ 3. Factors
_____ 4. Fraction
_____ 5. Improper fraction
_____ 6. Mixed number
_____ 7. Numerator
_____ 8. Percent
_____ 9. Proportion
_____ 10. Ratio
_____ 11. Reciprocal
_____ 12. Word factors

COLUMN B

A. The divisor of a fraction written in the bottom half of a common fraction

B. A part of a whole containing a numerator and a denominator

C. A portion of a whole divided into 100 parts

D. Fractions with the numerator larger than the denominator

E. A fraction with the numerator smaller than the denominator

F. Any numbers multiplied together to form a product

G. Fractions preceded by a whole number

H. The inverse of a fraction

I. The top portion of a fraction

J. Two ratios that are equal to each other

K. The units used in a mathematical term

L. A comparison of two amounts that represent a constant relationship between values

II. MATCH THE FOLLOWING

Match the term from Column A with the correct definition from Column B.

COLUMN A

_____ 1. Biological standard unit
_____ 2. Dosage
_____ 3. Nomogram
_____ 4. Division line
_____ 5. 24-hour clock
_____ 6. 2 pints (32 fluidounces)
_____ 7. 60 minims

COLUMN B

A. The amount of medication to be taken at a specific time

B. One quart

C. A chart made of multiple scales arranged so that use of a straightedge to connect known values can determine an unknown value at the point of intersection

D. A specific amount of a biologically active substance that is used pharmacologically or therapeutically

E. Separates the numerator from the denominator

F. Time keeping method in which the day runs from midnight to midnight and is divided into 24 hours, numbered 0 to 23

G. One fluidrachm or fluidram

III. MULTIPLE CHOICE

Circle the letter of the best answer.

1. You have reconstituted a 5,000 unit vial of a medication with 10 ml of diluent. How many units will you be administering if you give 2 ml?

   a. 500 units
   b. 1,000 units
   c. 1,500 units
   d. 2,000 units

2. You want to give 30 units of insulin using 100-U insulin and a tuberculin syringe. How many milliliters is this?

   a. 0.3ml
   b. 0.5ml
   c. 0.8ml
   d. 0.1ml

3. Calculate the BSA for a child who weighs 20 kg and whose height is 80 cm. The answer is

   a. 0.44 m².
   b. 0.66 m².
   c. 0.15 m².
   d. 1.3 m².

4. The dosage prescribed for a medication is 0.10 mg/kg. How many milligrams should be prescribed for a patient weighing 150 lbs?

   a. 2.3 mg
   b. 4.8 mg
   c. 5.3 mg
   d. 6.8 mg

5. The recommended dosage of a medication for a child is 2 mg/kg. How many milligrams should a child weighing 50 lbs is given?

   a. 10 mg
   b. 25 mg

   c. 45 mg
   d. 60 mg

6. You want to convert 130°F to C. The correct answer is

   a. 30°C.
   b. 45°C.
   c. 50°C.
   d. 54°C.

7. If a drug costs $10 per oz (avoir), what is the cost of two drams?

   a. $2.74
   b. $2.85
   c. $3.00
   d. $3.21

8. One liter equals

   a. 0.001 kiloliter.
   b. 0.01 kiloliter.
   c. 0.1 kiloliter.
   d. 0.0001 kiloliter.

9. When 75% is converted to a decimal, the answer is

   a. 7.5.
   b. 0.075
   c. 0.75
   d. 75

10. A patient is to receive a dose of medication at 4:00 pm today. How would the time be documented on the medication administration record?

   a. 1400
   b. 1500
   c. 1600
   d. 1800

IV. RECALL FACTS

Indicate which of the following statements are facts with an F. If the statement is not a fact, leave the line blank.

ABOUT MATH BASICS

_____ 1. The number 1/2 is an improper fraction.

_____ 2. The number 4 2/3 is a mixed number.

_____ 3. The number 3/4 is the reciprocal of 4/3.

_____ 4. The number 5 is a common denominator of 10 and 16.

_____ 5. 2/6 X 3/4 = 6/24.

_____ 6. 5.61 + 2.13 = 7.74.

ABOUT APOTHECARY MEASUREMENT TERMS
LABEL FLUID MEASUREMENTS WITH F AND WEIGHT MEASUREMENTS WITH W.

_____ 1. Minim

_____ 2. Grain

_____ 3. Fluidrachms

_____ 4. Scruple

_____ 5. Drachm

_____ 6. Ounce

V. FILL IN THE BLANKS

Fill in the blanks using figures/terms from the list below.

C = 5/9 (F-32)   1500   3/4   13/15   1/4   19/3   245.19   1 gram   9/5   1000 grams

1. _____ is the conversion formula from Fahrenheit to Celsius.

2. One kilogram equals _____.

3. _____ is equivalent to 3:00 PM

4. 1000 milligrams (mg) equals

   _____.

5. The reciprocal number of 5/9 is _____.

6. When 120/160 is reduced to lowest terms, the

   answer is _____.

7. When $6\frac{1}{3}$ is converted to an improper fraction,

   the answer is _____.

8. When 2/3 and 1/5 are added together, the answer

   is _____.

9. When 2/3 and 3/8 are multiplied, the answer is

   _____.

10. When 23.69 is multiplied by 10.35, the answer is

   _____.

VI. LIST

List the requested number of items.

1. List the five steps involved in the basic dimensional analysis problem.

   a. _____

   b. _____

   c. _____

   d. _____

   e. _____

2. List three biologically active substances used pharmacologically or therapeutically that are measured in biological standard units.

   a. _____

   b. _____

   c. _____

3. List six apothecary measures of fluids.

   a. _____

   b. _____

   c. _____

   d. _____

   e. _____

   f. _____

4. List four apothecary measures of weight.

   a. _____

   b. _____

   c. _____

   d. _____

   e. _____

5. List the place values for the position of each number below.
   8,634,841.16 345

   a. (8) _____

   b. (6) _____

   c. (3) _____

   d. (4) _____

   e. (8) _____

   f. (4) _____

   g. (1) _____

   h. (1) _____

   i. (6) _____

   j. (3) _____

   k. (4) _____

   l. (5) _____

VII. CLINICAL APPLICATIONS

1. You are preparing to administer a liquid oral
   medication to a child. For this medication, 10 cc is
   equal to a 5 mg dose. The dose you are to administer
   is 7.5 mg. How many cc's should you give?

VIII. CASE STUDY

Mr. Jones has been prescribed a medication that is
dosed 10 mg/kg/d to be given in four divided doses. You
have the liquid medication and the label reads 1 mg/ml.
Mr. Jones weighs 220 pounds.

1. How much medication should he receive daily?

   a. 10 mg
   b. 100 mg
   c. 110 mg
   d. 2200 mg

2. How much should he receive per dose?

   a. 2.5 mg
   b. 25 mg
   c. 27.5 mg
   d. 550 mg

3. How much liquid will you need per dose?

   a. 2.5 ml
   b. 25 ml
   c. 27.5 ml
   d. 550 ml

4

Central Nervous System Stimulants

I. MATCH THE FOLLOWING

Match the generic CNS stimulant drug from Column A with the trade name of the drug from Column B.

COLUMN A

____ 1. dextroamphetamine
____ 2. atomoxetine
____ 3. caffeine
____ 4. modafinil
____ 5. doxapram HCL
____ 6. methamphetamine
____ 7. dexmethylphenidate
____ 8. methylphenidate HCl
____ 9. lisdexamfetamine dimesylate
____ 10. phentermine HCl
____ 11. phendimetrazine
____ 12. benzphetamine HCl

COLUMN B

A. Desoxyn
B. Provigil
C. Dopram
D. Focalin
E. Dexedrine
F. Strattera
G. Concerta
H. Cafcit
I. Didrex
J. Adipex-P
K. Vyvanse
L. Bontril

II. MATCH THE FOLLOWING

Match the CNS stimulant from Column A with the drug use from Column B.

COLUMN A

_____ 1. phentermine

_____ 2. doxapram HCl

_____ 3. methylphenidate

_____ 4. dexmethylphenidate

_____ 5. modafinil

_____ 6. methamphetamine

_____ 7. caffeine

COLUMN B

A. Drug-induced CNS depression

B. Obesity

C. ADHD

D. Narcolepsy, shift work sleep disorders

E. ADHD, narcolepsy

F. Fatigue, drowsiness

G. ADHD, exogenous obesity

III. TRUE OR FALSE

Indicate whether each statement is True (T) or False (F).

_____ 1. Analeptics are drugs that depress the respiratory center.

_____ 2. The action of doxapram is to increase the depth of respirations by stimulating receptors located in the carotid arteries and the upper aorta.

_____ 3. Phentermine and phendimetrazine are amphetamines.

_____ 4. Amphetamines and anorexiants may be abused and can result in addiction.

_____ 5. A child with ADHD, once medicated, never has its drug regimen interrupted.

IV. MULTIPLE CHOICE

Circle the letter of the best answer.

1. Central nervous system stimulants include _____.

   a. anticonvulsants
   b. anorexiants
   c. analeptics
   d. amphetamines
   e. Answers b, c, and d

2. Which of the following drugs are considered to be analeptics?

   a. Modafinil
   b. Caffeine
   c. Doxapram
   d. Phentermine
   e. Answers a, b, and c

3. A patient who is taking an amphetamine may have _____.

   a. an increase in blood pressure
   b. an increase in pulse rate
   c. a decrease in pulse rate
   d. appetite suppression
   e. All of the above

4. All of the following except _____ are uses of amphetamines.

   a. exogenous obesity
   b. ADHD
   c. stimulation of skeletal muscle
   d. narcolepsy
   e. None of the above

5. A common adverse reaction from short-term use of amphetamines and anorexiants is _____.

    a. drowsiness
    b. overstimulation of the CNS
    c. fever
    d. dry mouth
    e. None of the above

6. Amphetamines and anorexiants use _____.

    a. may result in tolerance to the drug
    b. may cause psychological dependence
    c. is recommended only for short-term use for the treatment of exogenous obesity
    d. Both a and c
    e. Answers a, b, and c

7. All of the following are adverse reactions to dexmethylphenidate except _____.

    a. nervousness
    b. insomnia
    c. loss of appetite
    d. liver failure

8. All of the following are true about neurons except _____.

    a. they are the functional cells of the nervous system
    b. each neuron is made up of a soma, a dendrites, and an axon
    c. neurons conduct impulses to the spinal cord and brain
    d. neurons do not carry impulses from the CNS to the body's muscles and glands

9. Synapses

    a. prevent information from passing from one cell to another.
    b. link neurons.
    c. are responsible for the peripheral nervous system activities.
    d. cause narcolepsy.

10. Narcolepsy is

    a. a disorder causing an uncontrollable desire to sleep during normal waking hours.
    b. a disorder manifested by a short attention span.
    c. treated by using amphetamines.
    d. Both a and c

11. Attention deficit hyperactivity disorder is manifested by _____.

    a. a short attention span
    b. hyperactivity
    c. impulsiveness
    d. emotional lability
    e. All of the above

12. Anorexiants are used for _____.

    a. treating ADHD
    b. suppressing the appetite
    c. treating narcolepsy
    d. treating blood clots

13. Doxapram is used for _____.

    a. treating drug-induced CNS depression
    b. temporarily treating respiratory depression in patients with chronic pulmonary disease
    c. treating respiratory depression from anesthesia in the postanesthesia period
    d. All of the above

14. The effects of amphetamines on ADHD include _____.

    a. reduction of motor restlessness
    b. increased mental alertness
    c. elevated mood
    d. reduced feelings of fatigue
    e. All of the above

15. Adverse effects of central nervous system stimulants on older adults may include _____.

    a. excessive anxiety
    b. nervousness
    c. insomnia
    d. mental confusion
    e. All of the above

V. RECALL FACTS

Indicate which of the following statements are facts with an F. If the statement is not a fact, leave the line blank.

ABOUT PATIENTS IN WHOM CNS STIMULANTS ARE CONTRAINDICATED

_____ 1. Those with a known hypersensitivity

_____ 2. Those with severe hypertension

_____ 3. Within 2 weeks of receiving an MAOI

_____ 4. Guanethidine users

_____ 5. Tricyclic antidepressant users

_____ 6. Pregnant women

_____ 7. Newborns

_____ 8. Stroke victims

_____ 9. Those with convulsive states

_____ 10. Those with glaucoma

_____ 11. Those with hyperthyroidism

_____ 12. Those with head injuries

ABOUT MANAGING ADVERSE REACTIONS OF CNS STIMULANTS

_____ 1. To decrease insomnia, patients should take the drug early in the day.

_____ 2. Napping will reduce insomnia.

_____ 3. Using coffee, tea, or cola drinks will not affect the patient.

_____ 4. Increase the dosage if tolerance develops.

_____ 5. Cardiovascular disorders in elderly patients may be worsened while taking CNS stimulants therefore these patients should be monitored carefully.

VI. FILL IN THE BLANKS

Fill in the blanks using words from the list below.

phendimetrazine   amphetamines   analeptics   newborns   modafinil
anorexiants   narcolepsy   ADHD   insomnia   doxapram

1. _____ is believed to treat narcolepsy by increasing the alpha activity of the brain.

2. _____ are drugs used to suppress the appetite.

3. A common adverse reaction of the anorexiants is _____.

4. _____ are drugs used to stimulate the respiratory center.

5. _____ is a disorder causing an uncontrollable desire to sleep during normal waking hours.

6. _____ is a drug used to increase the depth of respirations.

7. Treatment of exogenous obesity may include a prescription for _____.

8. _____ should not be given central nervous system stimulants.

9. _____ are contraindicated in patients with glaucoma.

10. It is beneficial for a parent to write a daily summary of the child's behavior with _____.

VII. LIST

List the requested number of items.

1. List the three parts of a neuron.

    a. _____

    b. _____

    c. _____

2. List the three functions of neurons.

    a. _____

    b. _____

    c. _____

3. List six facts about caffeine.

    a. _____

    b. _____

    c. _____

    d. _____

    e. _____

    f. _____

4. List the three categories of CNS stimulants covered in this chapter.

    a. _____

    b. _____

    c. _____

5. List four manifestations of attention deficit disorder.

    a. _____

    b. _____

    c. _____

    d. _____

6. List four neurohormones (neurotransmitters) of the central nervous system.

    a. _____

    b. _____

    c. _____

    d. _____

7. List seven drugs used for ADHD.

    a. _____

    b. _____

    c. _____

    d. _____

    e. _____

    f. _____

    g. _____

8. List five drugs used for obesity.

    a. _____

    b. _____

    c. _____

    d. _____

    e. _____

9. List six adverse effects of anorexiants.

    a. _____

    b. _____

    c. _____

    d. _____

    e. _____

    f. _____

10. List six important elements of patient care when a CNS stimulant is given for respiratory depression.

    a. _____

    b. _____

    c. _____

    d. _____

    e. _____

    f. _____

VIII. CLINICAL APPLICATIONS

1. A child with ADHD has been prescribed
   a CNS stimulant. What information should
   the parent told about caring for the child while
   on this medication?

IX. CASE STUDY

Mary F., age 20 and a college student, has been diagnosed with narcolepsy. She has had problems with falling asleep while driving and with staying awake during
her classes. The physician has prescribed a medication
for Mary to take.

1. The drug most likely prescribed was
   a. modafinil.
   b. dexmethylphenidate.
   c. methamphetamine.
   d. benzphetamine HCl.

2. The drug prescribed for Mary is thought to
   a. decrease the delta-, theta-, and beta-activity.
   b. reduce the number of sleepiness episodes.
   c. increase the alpha activity in the brain.
   d. bind to dopamine reuptake carrier sites.
   e. All of the above

3. Adverse effects of the medication prescribed for
   Mary include
   a. anxiety.
   b. back pain.
   c. dyspepsia.
   d. nausea.
   e. All of the above

4. Mary's health care provider has recommended that
   she should do the following: _____.
   a. keep a record of the number of times per day
      that periods of sleepiness occur, and bring this
      record to each office visit
   b. take this drug on a regular schedule as she has
      epilepsy also
   c. refrain from any physical activity
   d. operate as much equipment as possible to test
      the effects of the drug

5

Anticonvulsants and Antiparkinsonism Drugs

I. MATCH THE FOLLOWING

Match the term from Column A with the correct definition from Column B.

COLUMN A

____ 1. Choreiform movements

____ 2. Dystonic movements

____ 3. Epilepsy

____ 4. Jacksonian seizure

____ 5. Psychomotor seizures

____ 6. Status epilepticus

____ 7. Tonic-clonic seizures

COLUMN B

A. An emergency situation characterized by continual seizure activity with no interruptions

B. A focal seizure that begins with uncontrolled stiffening or jerking of a part of the body, such as the finger, mouth, hand, or foot, that may progress to a generalized seizure

C. A permanent, recurrent seizure disorder

D. An alternate contraction and relaxation of muscles, a loss of consciousness, and abnormal behavior

E. The involuntary twitching of the limbs or the facial muscles

F. A seizure that may involve an aura with perceptual alterations, such as hallucinations or a strong sense of fear; most often occurs in children through adolescence

G. Muscular spasms most often affecting the tongue, jaw, eyes, and neck

II. MATCH THE FOLLOWING

Match the anticonvulsant generic drug from Column A with the drug use from Column B.

COLUMN A

____ 1. phenobarbital sodium

____ 2. clorazepate

____ 3. ethotoin

____ 4. ethosuximide

____ 5. vigabatrin

____ 6. oxcarbazepine

____ 7. primidone

____ 8. valproic acid

COLUMN B

A. Status epilepticus

B. Absence seizures

C. Tonic-clonic seizures, psychomotor seizures

D. Partial seizures

E. Refractory complex partial seizures

F. Epilepsy

G. Grand mal seizures

H. Absence seizures, complex partial seizures

III. MATCH THE FOLLOWING

Match the generic antiparkinsonism drug from Column A with the trade name of the drug from Column B.

COLUMN A

____ 1. entacapone
____ 2. benztropine mesylate
____ 3. rasagiline
____ 4. selegiline
____ 5. apomorphine
____ 6. carbidopa
____ 7. diphenhydramine
____ 8. pramipexole
____ 9. carbidopa/levodopa
____ 10. ropinirole HCl
____ 11. tolcapone
____ 12. bromocriptine

COLUMN B

A. Azilect
B. Benadryl
C. Cogentin
D. Lodosyn
E. Emsam
F. Apokyn
G. Mirapex
H. Parlodel
I. Requip
J. Sinemet
K. Comtan
L. Tasmar

IV. TRUE OR FALSE

Indicate whether each statement is True (T) or False (F).

____ 1. All seizure disorders have a known cause.

____ 2. The on–off phenomenon that can occur in patients taking levodopa may be managed by simply abruptly stopping all medications.

____ 3. Most anticonvulsants have specific uses and are used in the treatment of specific types of seizure disorders.

____ 4. Anticonvulsants work by increasing the excitability of the brain, thereby reducing the intensity and frequency of neural stimulation.

____ 5. Diazepam is commonly given to patients experiencing status epilepticus.

____ 6. A potentially fatal rash may occur in patients taking lamotrigine.

____ 7. Phenytoin is contraindicated in patients with certain cardiac problems and during pregnancy and lactation.

____ 8. Patients with bone marrow depression can be given succinimide as long as the dosage is low.

____ 9. Antiparkinsonism drugs are used to relieve the symptoms, not cure, Parkinson disease.

____ 10. Oral dopamine is able to cross the blood–brain barrier and therefore is the most effective treatment for Parkinson disease.

____ 11. Adverse reactions with levodopa and carbidopa in the early stages of treatment are not usually a problem.

V. MULTIPLE CHOICE

Circle the letter of the best answer.

1. All of the following are true about partial seizures except what?
   a. It can cause generalized seizures
   b. It arise from a localized area of the brain
   c. It include simple seizures, Jacksonian seizures, and psychomotor seizures
   d. It has a particular stimulus
   e. It can cause specific symptoms

2. Dosages of anticonvulsants ____.
   a. may be adjusted during times of stress or illness
   b. are often adjusted with increases or decreases during the initial period of treatment
   c. are always constant so as not to confuse the patient
   d. are only taken alone; combination therapy has not proven to be effective
   e. Both a and b

3. Adverse reactions of barbiturates can include
   _____.
   a. sedation
   b. agitation
   c. nausea
   d. hypersensitivity rash
   e. All of the above

4. Hydantoin's adverse reactions can include _____.
   a. nystagmus
   b. ataxia
   c. gingival hyperplasia
   d. blood dyscrasias
   e. All of the above

5. Succinimides _____.
   a. have frequent gastrointestinal symptoms
   b. rarely produce toxic effects
   c. can produce a potentially fatal rash
   d. may produce hematological changes
   e. Both a and d

6. In whom should barbiturates be either contraindicated or used with precaution?
   a. Hyperactive children
   b. Patients with pulmonary disease
   c. Patients with neurological disorders
   d. Patients with a known hypersensitivity to the drug
   e. All of the above

7. Hydantoins are contraindicated or used with
   caution in patients' _____.
   a. who are pregnant or lactating
   b. who have a known hypersensitivity to the drug
   c. who have eye disorders
   d. who have liver, kidney, or neurological
      disorders
   e. Answers a, b, and d

8. All of the following are classified as antiparkinsonism drugs except what?
   a. Dopamine receptor agonists
   b. Acetylcholinesterase inhibitors
   c. COMT inhibitors
   d. Anticholinergic drugs
   e. Dopaminergic drugs

9. Dopamine receptor agonists are contraindicated
   with, which of the following?
   a. Known hypersensitivity
   b. Severe ischemic heart disease
   c. Peripheral vascular disease
   d. All of the above

10. Choreiform and dystonic movements are the most
    serious and frequent adverse reactions seen with
    _____.
    a. carbidopa
    b. amantadine
    c. dopamine
    d. levodopa
    e. anticholinergics

11. Adverse reactions to anticholinergic drugs com-
    monly include dry mouth, blurred vision, dizzi-
    ness, and _____.
    a. nausea
    b. nervousness
    c. hiccoughs
    d. Both a and b
    e. All of the above

12. Patients older than 60 years of age who are taking
    anticholinergics _____.
    a. require higher doses of the drugs
    b. frequently develop increased sensitivity
    c. commonly become less confused
    d. All of the above

13. COMT inhibitors are thought to act by _____.
    a. stimulating dopamine release
    b. inhibiting acetylcholinesterase
    c. blocking an enzyme that eliminates dopamine
    d. blocking levodopa
    e. Both b and d

14. Dopamine receptor agonists' _____.
    a. are thought to mimic the effects of dopamine
       in the brain
    b. are used to treat the signs and symptoms of
       Parkinson's disease
    c. have common adverse reactions of nausea,
       dizziness, and postural hypotension
    d. should not be given to patients with ischemic
       heart disease
    e. All of the above

15. Adverse reactions associated with antiparkinson-
    ism drugs that can be managed by the health
    care provider to increase the comfort level of the
    patient include all of the following except _____.
    a. dry mouth
    b. urinary incontinence
    c. visual difficulties
    d. GI disturbances
    e. difficulty walking

VI. RECALL FACTS

Indicate which of the following statements are facts with an F. If the statement is not a fact, leave the line blank.

ABOUT MANAGING ADVERSE REACTIONS OF ANTICONVULSANTS

____ 1. Oral anticonvulsants are always taken on an empty stomach.

____ 2. The patient's ability to swallow should be checked before taking any drug.

____ 3. Precautions against injuries caused by seizures are needed until control is established.

____ 4. Drowsiness usually decreases with continued use of the drug.

____ 5. Barbiturates may produce excitement, depression, and confusion in older adults.

____ 6. Diazepam is given in standard dosages to elderly patients with no difficulties.

ABOUT PATIENT MANAGEMENT ISSUES WITH ANTIPARKINSONISM DRUGS

____ 1. Some patient histories may need to be obtained from the family members.

____ 2. The patient's neurological status needs to be established before drug therapy is started.

____ 3. With Parkinson disease, the health care provider is only concerned with monitoring drug therapy.

____ 4. Hallucination incidence with antiparkinsonism drugs appears to increase with age.

ABOUT ANTICONVULSANT MANAGEMENT ISSUES

____ 1. Anticonvulsant can cure epilepsy.

____ 2. The dosage of an anticonvulsant is frequently adjusted during the initial treatment period.

____ 3. Only one anticonvulsant is prescribed at a time.

____ 4. Regular testing for drug levels is done to monitor toxicity.

____ 5. Abrupt discontinuation of an anticonvulsant can result in status epilepticus.

____ 6. To discontinue an anticonvulsant, gradual withdrawal of the dosage should occur.

VII. FILL IN THE BLANKS

Fill in the blanks using words from the list below.

anticholinergic drugs   dystonic movements   drowsiness   anticonvulsants   choreiform movements
on–off phenomenon   tolcapone   additive   convulsion   dopamine   acetylcholine

1. A(n) _____ is essentially the same thing as a seizure.

2. Succinimides, barbiturates, benzodiazepines, and hydantoins are the four types of drugs used as _____.

3. _____ is the most common adverse reaction of diazepam.

4. The use of any of the four types of anticonvulsants with other CNS depressants can result in a(n) _____ CNS depressant effect.

5. _____ are muscular spasms most often affecting the tongue, jaw, eyes, and neck.

6. _____ are used as adjunctive therapy in all forms of parkinsonism.

7. Liver failure is a severe and potentially fatal adverse reaction that can occur with _____ administration.

8. Parkinson's disease is a progressive, degenerative disorder of the CNS thought to be caused by a decrease in _____ and an excess of _____ 5F.

9. _____ are involuntary muscular twitching of the limbs or the facial muscles.

10. With _____ a patient may suddenly alternate between improved clinical status and loss of therapeutic effect.

VIII. LIST

List the requested number of items.

1. List three situations in which levodopa is contraindicated.

    a. _____

    b. _____

    c. _____

2. List six drugs that interact with phenytoin.

    a. _____

    b. _____

    c. _____

    d. _____

    e. _____

    f. _____

3. List the four categories of antiparkinsonism drugs.

    a. _____

    b. _____

    c. _____

    d. _____

4. List seven types of patients in which benzodiazepines are either contraindicated or used with precaution.

    a. _____

    b. _____

    c. _____

    d. _____

    e. _____

    f. _____

    g. _____

5. List the five signs of phenytoin toxicity.

    a. _____

    b. _____

    c. _____

    d. _____

    e. _____

6. List the three types of partial or focal seizures.

    a. _____

    b. _____

    c. _____

7. List the three types of generalized seizures.

    a. _____

    b. _____

    c. _____

8. List eight symptoms of Parkinsonism.

    a. _____

    b. _____

    c. _____

    d. _____

    e. _____

    f. _____

    g. _____

    h. _____

9. List five adverse reactions of dopaminergic drugs.

    a. _____

    b. _____

    c. _____

    d. _____

    e. _____

10. List the three dopamine receptor agonist drugs.

    a. _____

    b. _____

    c. _____

IX. CLINICAL APPLICATIONS

1. A 30-year-old female coworker has been pre-scribed a hydantoin for her seizure disorder. The health care provider has asked you to go over some of the key points that she should know about taking this drug.

X. CASE STUDY

Mr. S., who was recently diagnosed with Parkinson's disease, has just been started on carbidopa/levodopa/entacapone. You are instructing him and his family about the drug, care, precautions, and possible adverse effects related to taking the drug.

1. The most common adverse effect of this medication is
   a. dry mouth.
   b. dyskinesias.
   c. urinary retention.
   d. tachycardia.

2. Dyskinesias include which of the following?
   a. Choreiform movements
   b. Dystonic movements
   c. Jacksonian seizures
   d. Both a and b

3. One of the effects of long-term levodopa treatment may be the
   a. on–off phenomenon.
   b. gingival hyperplasia.
   c. absence seizures.
   d. blood dyscrasias.

4. Recommendations to relieve the dry mouth associated with this drug include which of the following?
   a. Offering frequent sips of water
   b. Offering ice chips
   c. Sucking hard candy
   d. All of the above

6

Cholinesterase Inhibitors

I. MATCH THE FOLLOWING

Match the term from Column A with the correct definition from Column B.

COLUMN A

____ 1. Acetylcholine

____ 2. Alzheimer disease

____ 3. Alanine aminotransferase (ALT)

____ 4. Anorexia

____ 5. Dementia

____ 6. Cholinesterase inhibitors

____ 7. Hepatotoxic

COLUMN B

A. Capable of producing liver damage

B. A diminished appetite

C. A decrease in cognitive functioning

D. A natural chemical in the brain that is required for memory and thinking

E. A disease of the elderly causing progressive deterioration of mental and physical abilities

F. Drugs used to treat Alzheimer disease

G. An enzyme found predominately in the liver; high levels may indicate liver damage

II. MATCH THE FOLLOWING

Match the generic cholinesterase inhibitor drug from Column A with the trade name from Column B.

COLUMN A

____ 1. galantamine hydrobromide

____ 2. rivastigmine tartrate

____ 3. donepezil HCl

____ 4. tacrine HCl

COLUMN B

A. Aricept

B. Razadyne

C. Exelon

D. Cognex

III. MATCH THE FOLLOWING

Match the drug from Column A with the known drug interactions effect from Column B. You may use an answer more than once.

COLUMN A

____ 1. Anticholinergic drugs

____ 2. theophylline

____ 3. succinylcholine

____ 4. Cholinergic agonists

COLUMN B

A. Decrease in activity of the drug

B. Toxicity

C. Synergistic effect

IV. TRUE OR FALSE

Indicate whether each statement is True (T) or False (F).

____ 1. All patients respond equally well to the different cholinesterase inhibiting drugs on the market today. Therefore, it is rarely necessary to change a prescription once it is in use.

____ 2. The adverse reactions associated with the use of cholinesterase inhibiting drugs generally last only a few days and will diminish after the body adjusts to the medication.

____ 3. A patient's response to cholinesterase inhibitors is usually immediate and cures Alzheimer disease.

____ 4. Any treatment that slows the progression of symptoms in Alzheimer disease is considered successful.

V. MULTIPLE CHOICE

Circle the letter of the best answer.

1. Acetylcholine _____.
   a. is required for memory and thinking
   b. is slowly lost by Alzheimer patients
   c. is a neurohormone
   d. All of the above
   e. Both a and b

2. Cholinesterase inhibiting drugs _____.
   a. act to increase the level of acetylcholine in the CNS
   b. act by inhibiting the breakdown of acetylcholine
   c. act to slow the destruction of neurons and inhibit the breakdown of acetylcholine in the brain
   d. cure Alzheimer disease
   e. Answers a, b, and c

3. Cholinesterase inhibiting drugs are used to _____.
   a. help a patient fully recover from Alzheimer disease
   b. treat dementia associated with Alzheimer disease
   c. replace the loss of acetylcholine in the brain
   d. accelerate the breakdown of acetylcholine and speed the destruction of neurons
   e. None of the above

4. In general, cholinesterase inhibiting drugs _____.
   a. are effective for ,virtually, every patient
   b. may have a variable effectiveness on an individual basis
   c. effect only males
   d. exhibit a stimulating response

5. The drug with the fewest adverse reactions and considered to be the first drug of choice in treating Alzheimer disease is _____.
   a. Aricept
   b. Razadyne
   c. Exelon
   d. Cognex
   e. ALT

6. The drug _____ has the potential to be hepatotoxic and tends to cause more adverse reactions. It is also generally given in smaller and more frequent doses when it is prescribed.
   a. Aricept
   b. Razadyne
   c. Exelon
   d. Cognex
   e. ALT

7. The drug _____ appears to cause more adverse reactions such as nausea and severe vomiting.
   a. tacrine HCl
   b. galantamine hydrobromide
   c. donepezil HCl
   d. rivastigmine tartrate

8. If a patient exhibits adverse reactions _____.
   a. the caregiver should report the reactions to the health care provider
   b. the health care provider may discontinue the medication or lower the dosage
   c. the caregiver should ignore the reaction(s), knowing that they will disappear in a few days anyway
   d. the caregiver should change the dosage themselves
   e. Both a and b

9. Adverse reactions such as dizziness may place a patient at risk for injury. To minimize the risk of falling, the caregiver could _____.
   a. keep the patient in his or her room at all times
   b. restrain all patients
   c. allow the patient to roam at will
   d. provide a controlled, safe environment with assistive devices

10. A patient who is being medicated with tacrine should be monitored for _____.
    a. liver enzyme elevations
    b. increased ALT levels
    c. liver damage
    d. alanine aminotransferase level elevations
    e. All of the above

11. The use of cholinesterase inhibitor medication is contraindicated in which of the following patients?
    a. Patients who are pregnant
    b. Patients who are lactating
    c. Patients with a known hypersensitivity to drugs in the cholinesterase inhibitor medication
    d. All the above patients should not receive cholinesterase inhibitors
    e. Both b and c

12. Cholinesterase inhibiting drugs may be given with caution in which of the following patients?
    a. Patients with renal or hepatic disease
    b. Patients with bladder obstruction
    c. Patients with sick sinus syndrome or seizure disorders
    d. Patients with gastrointestinal bleeding, a history of ulcers, or asthma
    e. All the patients listed above should receive cholinesterase inhibitors with caution

13. Patients receiving cholinesterase inhibitors are assessed before and during therapy for improvement. Which aspects of the patient are assessed during therapy?
    a. Cognitive ability
    b. Functional ability
    c. Physical condition
    d. Only the cognitive and functional abilities are assessed
    e. Cognitive, functional, and physical conditions are assessed

VI. FILL IN THE BLANKS

Fill in the blanks using words from the list below

tacrine   ALT   several   mild   progressive
weight loss   eating problems

1. In the late stages of Alzheimer disease,

   _____ and _____

   are two major issues for patients and caregivers.

2. Alzheimer disease is a(n) _____

   disorder.

3. Adverse reactions associated with cholinesterase inhibitors are usually _____

   and generally do not last for more than

   _____ days.

4. Liver damage in patients taking

   _____ may be monitored with

   _____ levels.

VII. LIST

List the requested number of items

1. List four key points about taking cholinesterase inhibitors.

   a. _____

   b. _____

   c. _____

   d. _____

2. List three types of drugs used to treat Alzheimer disease.

   a. _____

   b. _____

   c. _____

VIII. CLINICAL APPLICATIONS

1. Mrs. P has been diagnosed with Alzheimer disease. Explain to her family what potential changes to her therapy may occur if she has a poor response to one therapy.

IX. CASE STUDY

Mr. G.'s Alzheimer disease has recently progressed. His family has found that he needs more care than in the recent past, and they have brought him to the health care provider for further evaluation.

1. What would be the symptoms suggesting the early dementia phase was present?
   a. He needs assistance in activities of daily living
   b. He is unable to recall important aspects of current life
   c. He has difficulty making choices
   d. He is still able to recall major facts related to family names, his name, family history, etc.
   e. All of the above

2. What might the health care provider do to change Mr. G.'s drug regimen?
   a. He may change dosages
   b. He may discontinue the current medication
   c. He may add a medication
   d. He may start the drug memantine
   e. Any of the above

3. What are the important care aspects for the family to be aware of?
   a. Mr. G. should be allowed to do live independently with frequent family visits if he chooses.
   b. Make sure that medications are taken exactly as directed
   c. Keep track of when the drugs are taken
   d. Ensure that the environment is safe
   e. All are true except a.

7

Psychiatric Drugs

I. MATCH THE FOLLOWING

Match the term from Column A with the correct definition from Column B.

COLUMN A

____ 1. Ataxia
____ 2. Bipolar disorder
____ 3. Dysphoric
____ 4. Dystonia
____ 5. Endogenous
____ 6. Photophobia
____ 7. Psychotic disorder
____ 8. Soporific
____ 9. Tardive dyskinesia
____ 10. Tolerance

COLUMN B

A. Extreme or exaggerated sadness, anxiety, or unhappiness
B. A psychiatric disorder characterized by severe mood swings from extreme hyperactivity to depression
C. Made within the body
D. Another term for a hypnotic drug
E. Facial grimacing and twisting of the neck into unnatural positions
F. Unsteady gait
G. A disorder characterized by extreme personality disorganization and a loss of contact with reality
H. Intolerance to light
I. A syndrome consisting of potentially irreversible, involuntary dyskinetic movements
J. Patient condition in which increasingly larger dosages are required to obtain the desired effect

II. MATCH THE FOLLOWING

Match the generic name of the sedative or hypnotic from Column A with the correct trade name from Column B.

COLUMN A

____ 1. amobarbital sodium
____ 2. zaleplon
____ 3. phenobarbital
____ 4. zolpidem tartrate
____ 5. pentobarbital sodium
____ 6. chloral hydrate
____ 7. flurazepam
____ 8. temazepam
____ 9. butabarbital
____ 10. mephobarbital

COLUMN B

A. Luminal
B. Butisol sodium
C. Sonata
D. Amytal sodium
E. Ambien
F. Dalmane
G. Restoril
H. Nembutal
I. Somnote
J. Mebaral

III. MATCH THE FOLLOWING

Match the antidepressant drug from Column A with the action from Column B.

COLUMN A

_____ 1. MAOIs
_____ 2. TCAs
_____ 3. SSRIs
_____ 4. Miscellaneous antidepressants

COLUMN B

A. Inhibit uptake of norepinephrine or serotonin at the presynaptic neuron
B. Not understood
C. Inhibit the uptake of serotonin
D. Inhibit the activity of monoamine oxidase

IV. MATCH THE FOLLOWING

Match the generic antipsychotic drug from Column A with the correct trade name from Column B.

COLUMN A

_____ 1. ziprasidone
_____ 2. risperidone
_____ 3. clozapine
_____ 4. prochlorperazine
_____ 5. haloperidol
_____ 6. pimozide
_____ 7. lithium
_____ 8. olanzapine
_____ 9. loxapine
_____ 10. quetiapine fumarate

COLUMN B

A. Lithobid
B. Haldol
C. Clozaril
D. Compazine
E. Orap
F. Risperdal
G. Seroquel
H. Geodon
I. Loxitane
J. Zyprexa

V. MATCH THE FOLLOWING

Indicate whether the drug listed from Column A is a sedative/hypnotic, antianxiety drug, or an antidepressant from Column B. You may use an answer more than once.

COLUMN A

_____ 1. alprazolam
_____ 2. flurazepam
_____ 3. triazolam
_____ 4. diazepam
_____ 5. trazodone
_____ 6. lorazepam
_____ 7. buspirone
_____ 8. fluoxetine
_____ 9. zolpidem
_____ 10. amitriptyline

COLUMN B

A. Sedative/hypnotic
B. Antidepressant
C. Antianxiety drug

VI. TRUE OR FALSE

Indicate whether each statement is True (T) or False (F).

_____ 1. Benzodiazepines are thought to have their tranquilizing action by potentiating the effects of gamma amino butyric acid.

_____ 2. The benzodiazepines and the nonbenzodiazepines have similar actions at the cellular level.

_____ 3. Antianxiety drugs must never be discontinued abruptly because severe withdrawal symptoms may occur.

_____ 4. If depressive symptoms occur daily or nearly every day for 2 weeks or more, the patient is said to have major depression.

_____ 5. Research indicates that antidepressants work by changing the brain's receptors for norepinephrine and serotonin.

_____ 6. Tricyclics are the drug of choice for treating depression in patients with preexisting cardiac disease or prostatic enlargement.

_____ 7. Most sedatives and hypnotics are controlled substances.

_____ 8. Supportive care is the main treatment of barbiturate toxicity.

_____ 9. Barbiturates are often administered for their strong analgesic action.

_____ 10. Patients should not drink alcohol while taking sedatives or hypnotics because there is an additive effect which increases the central nervous system depression.

_____ 11. Benzodiazepines are also called antianxiety drugs.

_____ 12. Sedatives and hypnotics include barbiturates and benzodiazepines.

_____ 13. Buspirone is used to treat anxiety, but it is not a controlled substance.

_____ 14. The use of barbiturates for longer than 2 weeks poses no physical or psychological dependence.

_____ 15. MAOIs are not widely used because of potential serious adverse reactions.

_____ 16. It is safe to use a miscellaneous antidepressant during pregnancy.

_____ 17. St. John's wort is useful for treating mild to moderate depression.

_____ 18. Reducing the dosage of the antipsychotic drug will usually reduce extrapyramidal effects.

_____ 19. Patients taking lithium should lower their fluid intake to keep a higher concentration of the drug in their system for a longer period.

_____ 20. Frequent assessments are necessary for patients taking antipsychotics over the long-term, because dosage adjustments may be necessary.

VII. MULTIPLE CHOICE

Circle the letter of the best answer.

1. Which of the following is not a group of barbiturates?
   a. Ultra-short-acting
   b. Short-acting
   c. Intermediate acting
   d. Long-acting
   e. Ultra-long-acting

2. Barbiturates generally act by _____.
   a. depressing the central nervous system
   b. causing mood alteration
   c. causing respiratory depression
   d. Both a and b
   e. Answers a, b, and c

3. Sedatives and hypnotics may be used _____.
   a. to treat anxiety
   b. to treat insomnia
   c. as part of a preoperative regimen
   d. to help manage an illness
   e. All of the above

4. Patient's respiratory function should be monitored _____ sedative or hypnotic use.
   a. before
   b. 30 minutes to 1 hour after
   c. frequently after 1 hour
   d. Both a and c
   e. Answers a, b, and c

5. Common adverse reactions with SSRIs include all of the following except _____.
   a. headache
   b. nervousness
   c. insomnia
   d. congestive heart failure
   e. nausea

6. Bupropion should be taken:
   a. regularly
   b. as needed
   c. once daily
   d. None of the above

7. St. John's wort has been used to treat _____.
   a. insect bites
   b. wounds and burns
   c. depression
   d. sleep disorders
   e. All of the above

8. Antipsychotic drugs are thought to act by _____.
   a. blocking the release of dopamine in the brain
   b. increasing the firing of neurons in areas of the brain
   c. inhibiting MAO
   d. stimulating the release of dopamine in the brain
   e. Both a and b

9. Chlorpromazine can be used _____.
   a. as an antipsychotic drug
   b. as an antiemetic drug
   c. to treat uncontrollable hiccoughs
   d. Both a and c
   e. Answers a, b, and c

10. All of the following are extrapyramidal effects except _____.
    a. akathisia
    b. Parkinson-like symptoms
    c. dystonia
    d. paranoid reactions
    e. None of the above

11. Tardive dyskinesia _____.
    a. has potentially irreversible, involuntary dyskinetic movements
    b. has no known treatment
    c. has a higher incidence in older women
    d. symptoms signal that the drug must be discontinued
    e. All of the above

12. Oral liquid concentrate antipsychotics are _____.
    a. light sensitive
    b. the cause of gastrointestinal adverse effects
    c. available in many flavors
    d. administered mixed in liquids such as juices and carbonated beverages
    e. Both a and d

13. Two types of antianxiety drugs are _____.
    a. sedatives and hypnotics
    b. barbiturates and nonbarbiturates
    c. MAOIs and COMTs
    d. benzodiazepines and nonbenzodiazepines
    e. None of the above

14. Which of the following antianxiety drugs is not a benzodiazepine?
    a. Alprazolam
    b. Hydroxyzine
    c. Diazepam
    d. Lorazepam
    e. Chlordiazepoxide

15. Antianxiety drugs _____.
    a. are not recommended for long-term therapy
    b. can result in drug dependence
    c. can also be used as sedatives
    d. generally do not cause severe adverse reactions
    e. All of the above

16. An elderly patient who is experiencing anxiety might be given _____ since it does not cause excessive sedation.
    a. buspirone
    b. clorazepate
    c. diazepam
    d. lorazepam
    e. oxazepam

17. When benzodiazepine toxicity occurs, which of the following drugs can be given as an antidote?
    a. Nonbenzodiazepines
    b. Flurazepam
    c. Flumazenil
    d. Lithium
    e. GABA

18. Other than in patients with a known hypersensitivity, in which conditions are antianxiety drugs contraindicated?
    a. Shock or coma
    b. Narrow angle glaucoma
    c. Depressed vital signs
    d. Acute alcoholic intoxication
    e. All of the above

19. In which of the following conditions are TCAs contraindicated?
    a. Recent myocardial infarction
    b. Pregnancy and lactation
    c. Patients about to receive or just had a myelogram
    d. Within 14 days of using an MAOI
    e. All of the above

VIII. RECALL FACTS

Indicate which of the following statements are facts with an F. If the statement is not a fact, leave the line blank.

ABOUT ADVERSE REACTIONS OF SEDATIVE AND HYPNOTICS

____ 1. The patient must be protected from harm with a safe environment when experiencing excitement or confusion.

____ 2. No additional doses of hypnotics may be given if a patient awakens during the night.

____ 3. If a patient experiences a drug hangover, the health care provider should be notified.

____ 4. Elderly patients are at a greater risk for oversedation, dizziness, and confusion.

ABOUT PATIENT MANAGEMENT ISSUES WITH ANTIANXIETY DRUGS

____ 1. Anxious patients generally have cool, pale skin.

____ 2. Only hospitalized patients may receive non-benzodiazepines.

____ 3. Prolonged therapy may lead to dependence.

____ 4. Parenteral administration is the safest way for elderly or debilitated patients to receive antianxiety drugs.

ABOUT CONTRAINDICATIONS, PRECAUTIONS, AND INTERACTIONS OF ANTIPSYCHOTIC DRUGS

____ 1. Antipsychotics are contraindicated in pregnant or lactating women.

____ 2. Patients who have a hypersensitivity to tartrazine should not take lithium.

____ 3. Taking an antipsychotic drug with alcohol may result in additive CNS depression.

____ 4. Antipsychotics are used commonly in patients exposed to extreme heat or phosphorus insecticides.

____ 5. Clozapine works synergistically with other drugs that suppress the bone marrow.

IX. FILL IN THE BLANKS

Fill in the blanks using words from the list below.

drug dependency	anxiolytic drug	insomnia	tyramine	haloperidol
fatal reaction	St. John's wort	lithium	MAOIs	

1. A(n) _____ is used to treat anxiety.

2. _____ should be discontinued several weeks before surgery becasue of a potential for unpredictable reactions.

3. Food containing _____ can cause a serious hypertensive crisis when eaten by a patient taking an MAOI.

4. Melatonin's most significant use is for the short-term treatment of _____.

5. If sertraline is taken with an MAOI, a potentially _____ can occur.

6. Patients may not safely use _____ in conjunction with any other antidepressant.

7. _____ is an antimanic drug which seems to alter sodium transport in the nerve and muscle cells.

8. Neuroleptic malignant syndrome, which is an adverse reaction of antipsychotic drugs, most often occurs in patients taking _____.

9. Sedatives and hypnotics are generally not given for longer than 2 weeks because of potential _____.

X. LIST

List the requested number of items.

1. List the three types of psychotherapeutic drugs used to treat mental illness.

   a. _____

   b. _____

   c. _____

2. List four adverse reactions associated with the use of barbiturates as a sedative or hypnotic.

   a. _____

   b. _____

   c. _____

   d. _____

3. List four types of patients in which sedative or hypnotic administration is contraindicated.

   a. _____

   b. _____

   c. _____

   d. _____

4. List three symptoms that would indicate to the health care provider that a sedative or hypnotic should be withheld.

   a. _____

   b. _____

   c. _____

5. List three facts about adverse effects of clozapine.

   a. _____

   b. _____

   c. _____

6. List five symptoms of a major depressive episode.

   a. _____

   b. _____

   c. _____

   d. _____

   e. _____

7. List the two most common adverse reactions of TCAs.

   a. _____

   b. _____

8. List the four conditions in which the use of MAOIs is contraindicated.

   a. _____

   b. _____

   c. _____

   d. _____

9. List the three drugs used to treat schizophrenia.

   a. _____

   b. _____

   c. _____

10. List three important adverse reactions of antipsychotics.

    a. _____

    b. _____

    c. _____

XI. CLINICAL APPLICATIONS

1. Miss K has decided on her own that after 6 weeks of treatment with a barbiturate that she no longer needs to take the medication. What are some of the symptoms that Miss K may experience as she goes through withdrawal of the drug?

2. The health care provider has asked you to explain to Mr. G some general information about taking his antidepressant medication. What key things should Mr. G know about using these drugs?

XII. CASE STUDY

Mr. D. is a winemaker and frequently entertains in his home. His health care provider has prescribed isocarboxazid for his depression. Treatment with an MAOI requires more complex management than that with other antidepressive agents.

1. What would be the most challenging aspect of taking a MAOI for Mr. D?
   a. Avoidance of foods containing tyramine
   b. The need to restrict fluids
   c. The need to increase exercise level
   d. None of the above

2. Mr. D. decided to have a little wine with dinner tonight. He does not feel well now. What are some of the symptoms he may be exhibiting?
   a. Headache
   b. Stiff neck
   c. Chest pain
   d. Nausea
   e. All of the above

3. Mrs. D. is concerned about her husband's symptoms. She takes his blood pressure and finds it is 200/110. What should she do?
   a. Relax, this is not a problem
   b. Notify the doctor, as a stroke or death may be possible
   c. Have more wine
   d. Put a cool cloth on his head

8

Analgesics and Antagonists

I. MATCH THE FOLLOWING

Match the term from Column A with the correct definition from Column B.

COLUMN A

_____ 1. Acute pain

_____ 2. Chronic pain

_____ 3. Antipyretic

_____ 4. Miosis

_____ 5. Opioids

_____ 6. Partial agonist

_____ 7. Salicylates

_____ 8. Tinnitus

COLUMN B

A. Pain that is of short duration and lasts less than 3 to 6 months

B. Pinpoint pupils

C. Narcotic analgesics obtained from the opium plant

D. A category of narcotic analgesic that binds to a receptor and causes a response, but the response is limited

E. Drugs that have analgesic, antipyretic, and anti-inflammatory effects

F. Ringing sound in the ear

G. A drug that reduces the elevated body temperature

H. Pain that lasts longer than 6 months

II. MATCH THE FOLLOWING

Match the generic salicylate or nonsalicylate from Column A with the trade name from Column B.

_____ 1. acetylsalicylic acid

_____ 2. acetaminophen

_____ 3. magnesium salicylate

_____ 4. buffered aspirin

COLUMN B

A. Bufferin

B. Extra Strength Doan's

C. Bayer

D. Tylenol

III. MATCH THE FOLLOWING

Match the generic NSAID from Column A with the trade name from Column B.

COLUMN A

_____ 1. celecoxib

_____ 2. ibuprofen

_____ 3. indomethacin

_____ 4. flurbiprofen

_____ 5. sulindac

_____ 6. naproxen

_____ 7. oxaprozin

_____ 8. meloxicam

_____ 9. diclofenac

_____ 10. fenoprofen

COLUMN B

A. Voltaren

B. Clinoril

C. Daypro

D. Celebrex

E. Mobic

F. Aleve

G. Indocin

H. Advil

I. Cataflam

J. Nalfon

IV. MATCH THE FOLLOWING

Match the generic narcotic analgesic from Column A with the trade name from Column B.

COLUMN A

_____ 1. meperidine

_____ 2. buprenorphine

_____ 3. hydromorphone

_____ 4. morphine sulfate

_____ 5. oxymorphone

_____ 6. oxycodone

_____ 7. alfentanil

_____ 8. fentanyl

_____ 9. methadone

_____ 10. butorphanol

COLUMN B

A. MS Contin

B. Dolophine

C. Sublimaze

D. OxyContin

E. Dilaudid

F. Stadol

G. Demerol

H. Opana

I. Alfenta

J. Buprenex

V. MATCH THE FOLLOWING

Match the trade name from Column A with the category of drug from Column B. You may use an answer more than once.

COLUMN A

_____ 1. Stadol

_____ 2. Alfenta

_____ 3. Talwin

_____ 4. Buprenex

_____ 5. Sublimaze

_____ 6. Stadol

_____ 7. Paregoric

_____ 8. Ultiva

COLUMN B

A. Agonist

B. Partial agonist

C. Agonist antagonist

VI. TRUE OR FALSE

Indicate whether each statement is True (T) or False (F).

_____ 1. Nonnarcotic analgesics are used to relieve pain and have the possibility of causing physical dependency.

_____ 2. The analgesic action of salicylates is owed to inhibition of prostaglandin.

_____ 3. Salicylism is caused by salicylate toxicity and is reversible with a reduction in dosage.

_____ 4. Tinnitus or impaired hearing caused by high blood salicylate levels will not disappear once the drug is discontinued.

_____ 5. Acetaminophen is the only nonsalicylate analgesic available in the United States.

_____ 6. Acetaminophen is widely used for its anti-inflammatory action.

_____ 7. Chronic alcoholics may safely take acetaminophen but should avoid NSAIDs.

_____ 8. The goal of acetaminophen therapy is relief of pain or reduction of elevated body temperature.

_____ 9. The NSAIDs have anti-inflammatory, anti-pyretic, and analgesic effects.

_____ 10. Patients may take salicylates or acetaminophen with food.

_____ 11. NSAIDs are nonnarcotic analgesics.

_____ 12. NSAIDs act by inhibiting the action of the enzyme cyclooxygenase.

_____ 13. When monitoring a patient taking an NSAID, the health care provider need only be notified if active bleeding occurs.

_____ 14. Age appears to increase the incidence of adverse reactions to NSAIDs.

_____ 15. Narcotic analgesics are classified as nonagonists, antagonists, or mixed agonists.

_____ 16. Morphine is the "model narcotic".

_____ 17. A major hazard of narcotic analgesic administration is respiratory depression.

_____ 18. Older adults may require a lower dosage of a narcotic analgesic.

_____ 19. In patient-controlled analgesia, it is easy for patients to accidentally overdose themselves.

_____ 20. OxyContin is an effective and safe drug for use in elderly patients because patients tend to have fewer adverse reactions than with morphine.

_____ 21. Naloxone can be used to reverse the effects of a narcotic if needed.

_____ 22. Patients using narcotics for severe pain often become addicted to the drug.

_____ 23. Naloxone is a narcotic antagonist that can abruptly reverse a narcotic depression.

_____ 24. Naltrexone use may inhibit the action of opioid antidiarrheals, antitussives, and analgesics.

VII. MULTIPLE CHOICE

Circle the letter of the best answer.

1. All of the following are types of nonnarcotic analgesic drugs except _____.
   a. salicylates
   b. partial agonists
   c. nonsalicylates
   d. nonsteroidal anti-inflammatory drugs
   e. All of the above

2. Salicylates have an _____ effect.
   a. analgesic
   b. antipyretic
   c. anesthetic
   d. anti-inflammatory
   e. Answers a, b, and d

3. Long-term salicylate use by older adults can lead to _____.
   a. addiction
   b. a reduction in the effectiveness of the drug
   c. gastrointestinal bleeding
   d. permanent hearing loss
   e. Reye's syndrome

4. Salicylates are contraindicated in all of the following patients except _____.
   a. patients receiving NSAID therapy
   b. patients receiving anticoagulant drugs
   c. patients with bleeding disorders
   d. children or teenagers with influenza or chickenpox
   e. patients receiving antineoplastic drugs

5. Acetaminophen _____.
   a. is the drug of choice for treating children with fever and flu-like symptoms
   b. has analgesic activities
   c. has antipyretic activities
   d. has anti-inflammatory activities
   e. Answers a, b, and c

6. Excessive doses of acetaminophen can cause _____.
   a. necrosis of the liver cells
   b. hemophilia
   c. gastrointestinal bleeding
   d. respiratory distress
   e. All of the above

7. Miss C has been taking acetaminophen for her osteoarthritis. Lately the drug has not been as effective, so Miss C has increased her dose to 6 g/day. As the health care worker taking care of her, what might you be watching for at this dose level?
   a. Nausea and vomiting
   b. Anorexia
   c. Abdominal pain
   d. Jaundice
   e. All of the above

8. What should a patient avoid while taking acetaminophen?
   a. Alcohol consumption
   b. Salicylates
   c. NSAIDs
   d. Both a and c
   e. All of the above

9. Miss G complains, about the fact, that before and after her dental surgery she is not to take her usual dose of salicylates for her arthritis. What might the health care provider suggests her to take; to relieve her pain and decrease the inflammation?
   a. Ibuprofen
   b. Acetaminophen
   c. Naproxen
   d. Mefenamic acid
   e. Answers a, c, and d

10. Celecoxib relieves pain without causing gastrointestinal upset because it selectively inhibits _____.
    a. prostaglandin synthesis
    b. cyclooxygenase-2 (COX-2)
    c. cyclooxygenase-1 (COX-1)
    d. both COX-1 and COX-2
    e. None of the above

11. Common adverse reactions of NSAIDs include _____.
    a. nausea and vomiting
    b. dizziness and vertigo
    c. cardiac arrhythmias
    d. skin rashes and ecchymoses
    e. All of the above

12. Of the following drugs, which is (are) available over-the-counter?
    a. Sulindac
    b. Celecoxib
    c. Naproxen
    d. Ibuprofen
    e. Both c and d

13. Patients who should not take any type of NSAID include those who are _____.
    a. allergic to porcine products
    b. sensitive to narcotics
    c. hypersensitive to aspirin
    d. experiencing flu-like symptoms
    e. have had a myocardial infarction

14. Narcotic analgesics _____.
    a. are used to manage moderate to severe acute and chronic pain
    b. lessen anxiety and sedation
    c. provide obstetrical analgesia
    d. relieve pain from a heart attack
    e. All of the above

15. In which of the following situations should the narcotic analgesic be withheld from a patient and the health care provider contacted immediately?
    a. An increase in the respiratory rate
    b. A significant decrease in the respiratory rate or a rate of 10 breaths/min or less
    c. A significant increase or decrease in the pulse rate
    d. A significant decrease in the blood pressure or a systolic pressure less than 100 mm Hg.
    e. Answers b, c, and d

16. Signs that a patient is developing a dependence on a narcotic include all of the following except _____.
    a. withdrawal symptoms
    b. frequent requests for the narcotic
    c. personality changes when the drug is not received
    d. anorexia and weight loss
    e. complaints of pain or failure of the drug to relieve pain

17. A patient who has been using or abusing narcotics may experience _____ when given an agonist–antagonist narcotic analgesic.

    a. a synergistic effect
    b. withdrawal symptoms
    c. no difference in effectiveness
    d. a decreased effectiveness
    e. None of the above

18. An increased risk of respiratory depression can occur with narcotic analgesic use _____.

    a. when they are administered too soon after barbiturate anesthesia
    b. in older adults
    c. in patients in a weakened state
    d. in debilitated patients
    e. All of the above

19. By which routes can morphine be administered?

    a. Orally and rectally
    b. Subcutaneously
    c. Intramuscularly
    d. Intravenously
    e. All of the above

20. Epidural administration of narcotic analgesics has all of the following advantages except _____.

    a. fewer adverse reactions
    b. lower total dosage of drug
    c. greater patient comfort
    d. more adverse reactions
    e. direct effect on opiate receptors

21. Naloxone _____.

    a. is used to prevent the effects of opiates in the treatment of narcotic-dependent patients
    b. can restore respiratory function in 1 to 2 minutes
    c. has no activity if no opiates have been taken
    d. can be used to diagnose a suspected opioid overdosage
    e. All of the above

22. All of the following statements about naltrexone are correct except one. Which is the exception?

    a. Naltrexone completely blocks the effects of IV opiates.
    b. Naltrexone is used to treat patients dependent on opioids.
    c. Naltrexone alone will keep patients in an opioid-free state.
    d. Patients being treated with naltrexone have usually been detoxified and are enrolled in a treatment program.
    e. If taking naltrexone on a scheduled basis, opiate will have no narcotic effect.

VIII. RECALL FACTS

Indicate which of the following statements are facts with an F. If the statement is not a fact, leave the line blank.

ABOUT USES FOR SALICYLATES

____ 1. Relief of mild to moderate pain

____ 2. Decreased risk of MI in certain patients

____ 3. Decreased risk of TIA or strokes caused by fibrin platelet emboli in men

____ 4. Relief of pain associated with cancer

____ 5. Relief of bacterial endotoxin tissue damage

____ 6. Reduction of elevated body temperature

____ 7. Treatment of inflammatory conditions

ABOUT ADVERSE REACTIONS CAUSED BY LONG-TERM USE OF ACETAMINOPHEN

____ 1. Hemolytic anemia

____ 2. Respiratory depression

____ 3. Hypoglycemia

____ 4. Skin eruptions or urticaria

____ 5. Hepatotoxicity

____ 6. Elevated blood pressure

ABOUT SYNTHETIC ANALGESICS

____ 1. Hydromorphone

____ 2. Methadone

____ 3. Oxymorphone

____ 4. Levorphanol

____ 5. Remifentanil

____ 6. Oxycodone

____ 7. Meperidine

ABOUT PATIENTS IN WHOM ALL NARCOTIC ANALGESICS ARE CONTRAINDICATED

____ 1. Osteoarthritis

____ 2. Known hypersensitivity

____ 3. Acute bronchial asthma

____ 4. Myocardial infarction

____ 5. Upper airway obstruction

____ 6. Head injury

____ 7. Increased intracranial pressure

____ 8. Recent dental surgery

____ 9. Convulsive disorders

____ 10. Renal or hepatic dysfunction

____ 11. Reye's syndrome

____ 12. Acute ulcerative colitis

IX. FILL IN THE BLANKS

Fill in the blanks using words from the list below. You may use a word more than once.

depressed	PRN	with	decrease	one
COX-2	COX-1	increase	fewer	greater
ibuprofen	potent	methadone	scheduled	agonist
agonist–antagonist	naproxen	inhibiting	celecoxib	lower

1. Aspirin has a(n) _____ anti-inflammatory effect and a(n) _____ effect on platelets than do other salicylates, and also has a(n) _____ inhibitory effect on prostaglandin synthesis.

2. Willow bark has _____ adverse reactions than salicylates.

3. Acetaminophen may _____ blood glucose values.

4. Patients should discontinue salicylate therapy at least _____ week(s) before any type of surgery.

5. To prevent gastric upset, patients may take salicylates or acetaminophen _____ food or water.

6. The anti-inflammatory effects of NSAIDs are due to the inhibition of _____, whereas the gastrointestinal adverse reactions are due to blocking of _____.

7. NSAIDs can prolong bleeding time and _____ the effects of anticoagulants, but can _____ the effects of antihypertensive drugs.

8. _____ is contraindicated in patients allergic to sulfonamides.

9. _____ and _____ increase the risk of lithium toxicity in patients taking both drugs.

10. An opioid used for the treatment and management of opiate dependency is _____.

11. Narcotic analgesic adverse reactions differ according to whether the narcotic acts as a(n) _____ or a(n) _____.

12. When adverse reactions to narcotic analgesics occur, the health care provider may _____ the dose in an effort to _____ the intensity of the reaction.

13. The cough reflex of a patient taking a narcotic may be _____.

14. Morphine, when used to treat chronic pain, such as in cancer, is not given on a _____ basis but on a _____ basis.

X. LIST

List the requested number of items.

1. List the three types of pain.

   a. _____

   b. _____

   c. _____

2. List the four examples of salicylates by trade name.

   a. _____

   b. _____

   c. _____

   d. _____

3. List six adverse reactions associated with salicylates.

   a. _____

   b. _____

   c. _____

   d. _____

   e. _____

   f. _____

4. List four conditions in which patients may find acetaminophen treatment useful.

   a. _____

   b. _____

   c. _____

   d. _____

5. List four uses of NSAIDs.

   a. _____

   b. _____

   c. _____

   d. _____

6. List the three receptors that are involved in the actions of narcotic analgesics.

   a. _____

   b. _____

   c. _____

7. List the six factors that determine the ability of a narcotic analgesic to relieve pain.

   a. _____

   b. _____

   c. _____

   d. _____

   e. _____

   f. _____

XI. CLINICAL APPLICATIONS

1. Mr. G will be taking an NSAID as part of his treatment program. What information should the health care provider make sure that Mr. G knows about these drugs?

2. Mrs. Z has had a surgical procedure and has been placed on a PCA infusion pump. What should Mrs. Z have been instructed about the pump before its use?

XII. CASE STUDY

Sue Jones, age 25, was admitted to the hospital to have a complex reconstruction of her jaw. Postoperatively she was sent to the intermediate care unit (IMC) so that she

could be observed more closely. Sue's pain medication, morphine, was being delivered via a PCA pump.

1. Sue was concerned that she might inadvertently push the medication button too often and receive too much medication. What would you tell her?

   a. "Don't worry, a little extra medication won't hurt you."
   b. "The pump does not allow too much to be given, as a time interval between doses is set (a lockout interval)."
   c. "Press the call light instead of the medication button and I'll come and push the medication button for you."
   d. All of the above

2. Sue was placed on a cardiac and respiratory monitor in the IMC. The monitor alarm sounded and

   the nurse quickly came into the room. The respiratory monitor displayed a rate of eight. What is the most likely cause for this?

   a. Respiratory depression from the morphine
   b. The monitor is not functioning properly
   c. Sue had just gone to sleep
   d. None of the above

3. What might the staff do to help prevent a recurrence of the alarm?

   a. Stop the morphine
   b. Increase the morphine dose
   c. Decrease the morphine dose
   d. Bring the emergency cart to the room

9

Anesthetic Drugs

I. MATCH THE FOLLOWING

Match the term from Column A with the correct definition from Column B.

COLUMN A

_____ 1. Analgesia
_____ 2. Anesthesia
_____ 3. Atelectasis
_____ 4. Conduction block
_____ 5. General anesthesia
_____ 6. Local anesthesia
_____ 7. Patency
_____ 8. Regional anesthesia

COLUMN B

A. Being open or exposed

B. Provision of a pain-free state for the entire body

C. Reduction of air in the lungs

D. Absence of pain

E. Anesthesia produced by injecting a local anesthetic around nerves to limit the pain signals sent to the brain

F. Provision of a pain-free state in a specific area

G. Type of regional anesthesia produced by injection of a local anesthetic into or near a nerve trunk

H. A loss of feeling or sensation

II. MATCH THE FOLLOWING

Match the type of anesthesia from Column A with the injection site from Column B.

COLUMN A

_____ 1. Topical
_____ 2. Local infiltration
_____ 3. Regional
_____ 4. Spinal
_____ 5. Epidural block
_____ 6. Transsacral block
_____ 7. Brachial plexus

COLUMN B

A. Subarachnoid space of the spinal cord (L2)

B. Into the brachial plexus

C. Epidural space at the level of sacrococcygeal notch

D. In tissues

E. The surface of the skin, open area, or mucous membrane

F. The space surrounding the dura of the spinal cord

G. Around nerves

III. MATCH THE FOLLOWING

Match the stage number of general surgical anesthesia from Column A with the description from Column B.

COLUMN A

_____ 1. Stage 1

_____ 2. Stage 2

_____ 3. Stage 3

_____ 4. Stage 4

COLUMN B

A. Surgical analgesia

B. Induction—lasts until the patient loses consciousness

C. Respiratory paralysis

D. Delirium and excitement

IV. MATCH THE FOLLOWING

Match the anesthetic drug listed from Column A with the correct anesthetic classification from Column B. You may use an answer more than once.

COLUMN A

_____ 1. lidocaine HCl

_____ 2. cisatracurium besylate

_____ 3. atracurium besylate

_____ 4. scopolamine

_____ 5. tetracaine HCl

_____ 6. fentanyl

_____ 7. diazepam

_____ 8. procaine HCl

_____ 9. vecuronium bromide

COLUMN B

A. Preanesthetic

B. Local anesthetic

C. Muscle relaxant used during general anesthesia

V. MATCH THE FOLLOWING

Match the type of anesthesia commonly used from Column A with the procedure listed from Column B. You may use an answer more than once.

COLUMN A

_____ 1. Topical

_____ 2. Local infiltration

_____ 3. Epidural block

_____ 4. Transsacral block

_____ 5. Brachial plexus block

COLUMN B

A. Hand surgery

B. Obstetrics

C. Desensitize skin for injection of local anesthesia

D. Tissue sample for biopsy

VI. TRUE OR FALSE

Indicate whether each statement is True (T) or False (F).

_____ 1. The two types of anesthesia are regional and spinal.

_____ 2. Spinal anesthesia and conduction blocks are two types of regional anesthesia.

_____ 3. A preanesthetic drug is only used before the administration of a general anesthetic.

_____ 4. A preanesthetic drug may be given up to 2 hours before surgery.

_____ 5. Cholinergic blocking drugs are used as pre-anesthetic drugs because they decrease the secretions of the upper respiratory tract.

_____ 6. During the administration of general anesthesia, reflexes such as the swallowing and gag reflex are lost.

_____ 7. IV and IM methods of administration are most commonly used for general anesthetics.

_____ 8. Anesthesia begins with the loss of consciousness.

_____ 9. Nitrous oxide is the most commonly used anesthetic gas.

_____ 10. Methohexital and thiopental do not produce analgesia.

VII. MULTIPLE CHOICE

Circle the letter of the best answer.

1. A patient receiving local anesthesia _____.
   a. never requires sedation
   b. often has no memory of the procedure
   c. has had many preanesthetic drugs
   d. is fully awake but does not feel pain in the area that has been anesthetized
   e. None of the above

2. Examples of conduction block anesthetics include all of the following except _____.
   a. epidural
   b. spinal
   c. transsacral
   d. brachial plexus
   e. Answers a, c, and d

3. Preparing a patient for local anesthesia may involve _____.
   a. an allergy history
   b. prepping the body area for the procedure
   c. giving the patient a sedative
   d. an explanation of the administration of the anesthetic
   e. All of the above

4. Which of the following can be used as preanesthetic drugs?
   a. Narcotics
   b. Cholinergic blocking drugs
   c. Antianxiety drugs
   d. Antiemetics
   e. All of the above

5. A general anesthetic produces _____.
   a. a pain-free state for the entire body
   b. a pain-free state for a part of the body
   c. a loss of consciousness
   d. Both a and c
   e. Answers a, b, and c

6. Which of the following drugs is a nonbarbiturate used for induction of anesthesia?
   a. etomidate
   b. ketamine
   c. midazolam
   d. ethylene
   e. isoflurane

7. During general anesthesia, a skeletal muscle relaxant, such as _____, may be used to facilitate intubation of the patient or relax skeletal muscles for surgical procedures.
   a. chlordiazepoxide
   b. pancuronium bromide
   c. morphine sulfate
   d. ropivacaine
   e. sevoflurane

8. Antiemetics are used to prevent _____ during the immediate postoperative recovery period.
   a. nausea and vomiting
   b. diarrhea and gastric upset
   c. vertigo
   d. drooling and coughing
   e. dry mouth and wheezing

9. Droperidol may be used _____.
   a. alone as a tranquilizer
   b. as an antiemetic in the immediate postanesthesia period
   c. as an induction drug
   d. as an adjunct to general anesthesia
   e. All of the above

10. The drug _____ is used for continuous sedation of intubated or respiratory-controlled patients in intensive care units.
    a. etomidate
    b. ketamine
    c. propofol
    d. midazolam
    e. ethylene

VIII. RECALL FACTS

Indicate which of the following statements are facts with an F. If the statement is not a fact, leave the line blank.

ABOUT DRUGS USED FOR INDUCTION AND MAINTENANCE OF ANESTHESIA

Which of the following are used for induction & mainte-nance of anesthesia

____ 1. cyclopropane

____ 2. enflurane

____ 3. nitrous oxide

____ 4. sevoflurane

____ 5. halothane

____ 6. propofol

____ 7. ethylene

____ 8. ketamine

____ 9. isoflurane

____ 10. midazolam

____ 11. desflurane

____ 12. remifentanil HCl

IX. FILL IN THE BLANKS

Fill in the blanks using words from the list below.

neuroleptanalgesia	inhaled anesthetic
thiopental	Innovar

etomidate	methohexital
explosive	decrease

1. Sublimaze and inapsine when used together as a single drug are called _____ .

2. Cyclopropane and ethylene when used mixed with oxygen are _____ .

3. Innovar results in _____ .

4. Sevoflurane is a(n) _____ .

5. _____ is a nonbarbiturate used for induction of anesthesia.

6. _____ and _____ are ultra–short-acting barbiturates that depress the CNS to produce hypnosis and anesthesia.

7. Cholinergic blocking drugs are used to _____ secretions of the upper respiratory tract.

X. LIST

List the requested number of items.

1. List four examples of a volatile liquid anesthetic.

a. _____

b. _____

c. _____

d. _____

2. List five uses of local anesthetics.

a. _____

b. _____

c. _____

d. _____

e. _____

3. List four reasons to use a preanesthetic drug.

a. _____

b. _____

c. _____

d. _____

4. List three factors that help determine the choice of anesthetic drug used for general anesthesia.

a. _____

b. _____

c. _____

XI. CLINICAL APPLICATIONS

1. The health care provider for whom you work has recommended surgery using general anesthesia for Mrs. Y's hysterectomy. Please explain to the patient the different stages of anesthesia she will undergo during this procedure.

XII. CASE STUDY

Mr. Jones is having general anesthesia for repair of his right rotator cuff. He is being given preanesthetic drugs prior to his procedure.

1. All of the following would be possible drugs that could be given except
   a. midazolam
   b. rocuronium bromide.
   c. fentanyl.
   d. droperidol.

2. The general anesthetic used for this procedure is methohexital sodium. The route of administration for this medication includes all of the following except
   a. rectal.
   b. IV.
   c. IM.
   d. inhalation.

3. The stages of anesthesia that should safely occur during Mr. Jones' anesthesia will include all of the following except
   a. analgesia.
   b. delirium.
   c. surgical analgesia.
   d. respiratory paralysis.

10

Antiemetic and Antivertigo Drugs

I. MATCH THE FOLLOWING

Match the term from Column A with the correct definition from Column B.

COLUMN A

_____ 1. Antiemetic

_____ 2. Nausea

_____ 3. Prophylaxis

_____ 4. Vertigo

_____ 5. Vestibular neuritis

_____ 6. Antivertigo

_____ 7. Emesis

_____ 8. Chemoreceptor trigger zone

COLUMN B

A. A drug used to treat or prevent nausea or vomiting

B. An unpleasant gastric sensation that usually preceding vomiting

C. An abnormal feeling of spinning or rotation motion that may occur with motion sickness and other disorders

D. Inflammation of the vestibular nerve to the inner ear

E. The expelled gastric contents

F. A drug or treatment designed for prevention of a condition or symptom

G. A drug used to treat or prevent vertigo

H. A group of nerve fibers in the brain, that when stimulated by chemicals, send impulses to the vomiting center of the brain

II. MATCH THE FOLLOWING

Match the generic name of the drug from Column A with the trade name from Column B.

COLUMN A

_____ 1. dolasetron

_____ 2. dimenhydrinate

_____ 3. diphenhydramine

_____ 4. trimethobenzamide

_____ 5. dronabinol

_____ 6. promethazine

_____ 7. prochlorperazine

_____ 8. ondansetron

_____ 9. meclizine

_____ 10. transdermal scopolamine

COLUMN B

A. Dramamine

B. Antivert

C. Phenergan

D. Compro

E. Zofran

F. Tigan

G. Marinol

H. Benadryl

I. Anzemet

J. Transderm-Scop

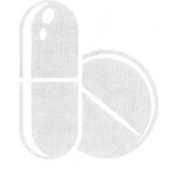

53

III. MATCH THE FOLLOWING

Match the drug from Column A with the contraindication, precaution, or interaction from Column B.

COLUMN A

____ 1. prochlorperazine

____ 2. promethazine

____ 3. trimethobenzamide

____ 4. antiemetics

____ 5. dimenhydrinate

____ 6. ondansetron

____ 7. ginger

COLUMN B

A. Bone marrow depression, blood dyscrasia, Parkinson's disease, severe liver disease

B. Patients with gallstones or hypertension

C. Hypertension, sleep apnea, epilepsy

D. Ototoxic drugs

E. Children with viral illnesses

F. Antacids

G. Rifampin

IV. TRUE OR FALSE

Indicate whether each statement is True (T) or False (F).

____ 1. An antivertigo drug is used to prevent nausea.

____ 2. Vomiting caused by drugs, radiation, or metabolic disorders usually occurs because of stimulation of the chemoreceptor trigger zone.

____ 3. Antiemetics are used to induce vomiting in cases of drug overdoses.

____ 4. The most common adverse reaction of antiemetic and antivertigo drugs is varying degrees of drowsiness.

____ 5. Antiemetics are not recommended during lactation or for uncomplicated vomiting in young children.

____ 6. Ginger is used to reduce nausea, vomiting, and indigestion.

____ 7. Patients who are being treated with antiemetic or antivertigo drugs have no alcohol restrictions.

____ 8. Driving should be avoided while taking antiemetic or antivertigo drugs.

____ 9. It is not a problem for patients to "share" their transdermal scopolamine patches while on a cruise because everyone is young and healthy.

V. MULTIPLE CHOICE

Circle the letter of the best answer.

1. A drug that would be more effective for vertigo associated with middle or inner ear surgery would probably act _____.

   a. by inhibiting the chemoreceptor trigger zone in the brain

   b. by depressing the vestibular apparatus of the inner ear

   c. by sending impulses to the vomiting center in the medulla

   d. by changing the patients electrolyte balance

   e. None of the above

2. Prophylactic antiemetics are commonly given to patients' _____.

   a. before surgery

   b. before antineoplastic drug administration

   c. with bacterial or viral infections

   d. before radiation therapy

   e. All of the above

3. Antivertigo drugs are commonly used _____.

   a. as an antiemetic

   b. to treat vertigo

   c. to treat motion sickness

   d. to prevent nausea and vomiting

   e. All of the above

4. Patients in whom antiemetic and antivertigo drugs are contraindicated include those _____.
   a. with a known hypersensitivity to the drugs
   b. in a coma
   c. with severe CNS depression
   d. Both a and b
   e. Answers a, b, and c

5. Antiemetic drugs may hamper the diagnosis of disorders such as _____.
   a. brain tumors
   b. appendicitis
   c. intestinal obstruction
   d. drug toxicity
   e. All of the above

VI. RECALL FACTS

Indicate which of the following statements are facts with an F. If the statement is not a fact, leave the line blank.

ABOUT PATIENT MANAGEMENT ISSUES FOR ANTIEMETICS AND ANTIVERTIGO DRUGS

____ 1. Dehydration is a serious concern in patients experiencing vomiting.

____ 2. Patients may need to be weighed daily or weekly if they experience prolonged or repeated episodes of vomiting.

____ 3. Patients experiencing vomiting after being given the oral form of an antiemetic drug should be given either a parenteral form or a rectal suppository form of antiemetic.

____ 4. Before starting drug therapy, vital signs should be taken.

____ 5. Elderly patients are at no higher risk for developing fluid and electrolyte disturbances caused by vomiting.

VII. FILL IN THE BLANKS

Fill in the blanks using words from the list below.

| additive | dehydration | diphenhydramine | antiemetics |
| vertigo | dimenhydrinate | ginger | antacids |

1. Elderly or chronically ill patients experiencing vomiting may develop _____ rapidly.

2. _____ may mask the signs and symptoms of ototoxicity when administered with ototoxic drugs.

3. Antiemetic and antivertigo drugs may have _____ effects when used with alcohol and other CNS depressants.

4. Antivertigo drugs are essentially the same as _____ .

5. A person experiencing _____ often has trouble walking.

6. _____ decrease the absorption of the antiemetics.

7. _____ is not recommended for morning sickness associated with pregnancy.

8. _____ is also used as an antihistamine.

VIII. LIST

List the requested number of items.

1. List the trade names of five antiemetic drugs that are used for patients receiving antineoplastic drug therapy.

   a. _____

   b. _____

   c. _____

   d. _____

   e. _____

2. List the generic names of three drugs used to treat motion sickness.

   a. _____

   b. _____

   c. _____

3. List three adverse effects of prochlorperazine.

   a. _____

   b. _____

   c. _____

4. List the six Pregnancy Category C antiemetics and antivertigo drugs.

   a. _____

   b. _____

   c. _____

   d. _____

   e. _____

   f. _____

IX. CLINICAL APPLICATIONS

1. Miss Q is getting married and planning a cruise for her honeymoon trip. She knows that she experiences motion sickness when she travels and has come to her health care provider to get a prescription to prevent this event from marring her honeymoon. What should Miss Q be aware of regarding the use of antivertigo drugs in general?

X. CASE STUDY

Mr. White, age 80, has been experiencing nausea and vomiting associated with the administration of chemotherapy for prostate cancer.

1. What are the special concerns we may have for Mr. White?

   a. Elderly patients who experience vomiting may have severe dehydration develop in a short time.
   b. He may develop fluid and electrolyte disturbances.
   c. We would treat him the same as any other patient experiencing vomiting.
   d. Both a and b

2. The staff is concerned that Mr. White may be dehydrated. All of the following are signs of dehydration except _____ .

   a. poor skin turgor
   b. dry mucous membranes
   c. decreased urinary output
   d. concentrated urine
   e. hypertension

3. All of the following are drugs that may be given for Mr. White's vomiting except _____ .

   a. Zofran
   b. Aloxi
   c. Dramamine
   d. Emend

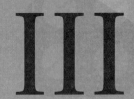

11

Adrenergic Drugs

I. MATCH THE FOLLOWING

Match the term from Column A with the correct definition from Column B.

COLUMN A

____ 1. Cardiac arrhythmia

____ 2. Neurotransmitter

____ 3. Orthostatic hypotension

____ 4. Acetyl choline

____ 5. Shock

____ 6. Vasopressor

____ 7. Peripheral nervous system

____ 8. Autonomic nervous system

COLUMN B

A. A life-threatening condition occurring when the supply of arterial blood flow and oxygen to the cells and tissues is inadequate

B. The branch of peripheral nervous system that controls the functions essential for survival

C. Irregular heartbeat

D. A drug that raises the blood pressure because it constricts blood vessels

E. A feeling of light-headedness and dizziness after suddenly changing from a lying to a sitting or a standing position

F. A neurotransmitter in the parasympathetic nervous system

G. All nerves outside the brain and spinal cord, connecting all parts of the body with the central nervous system

H. A chemical substance released at nerve ending to help transmit nerve impulses

II. MATCH THE FOLLOWING

Match the item from Column A with the correct definition from Column B.

COLUMN A

_____ 1. Central nervous system (CNS)

_____ 2. Peripheral nervous system (PNS)

_____ 3. Somatic nervous system (SNS)

_____ 4. Autonomic nervous system (ANS)

_____ 5. Parasympathetic nervous system

_____ 6. Sympathetic nervous system

COLUMN B

A. The branch of the PNS that controls the functions essential for life

B. The branch of the PNS that controls the sensation and voluntary movement

C. The branch of the ANS that regulates the expenditure of body energy

D. Consists of the brain and spinal cord

E. All nerves outside the brain and spinal cord

F. The branch of the ANS that helps to conserve body energy

III. MATCH THE FOLLOWING

Match the generic adrenergic drug from Column A with the trade name of the drug from Column B.

COLUMN A

_____ 1. dopamine

_____ 2. isoproterenol

_____ 3. midodrine

_____ 4. dobutamine

_____ 5. epinephrine

COLUMN B

A. ProAmatine

B. Dobutrex

C. Intropin

D. Isuprel

E. Adrenalin

IV. MATCH THE FOLLOWING

Match the adrenergic drug from Column A with the corresponding contraindication from Column B.

COLUMN A

_____ 1. isoproterenol

_____ 2. dopamine

_____ 3. epinephrine

_____ 4. norepinephrine

_____ 5. midodrine

COLUMN B

A. Narrow angle glaucoma

B. Severe organic heart disease

C. Pheochromocytoma

D. Tachyarrhythmias

E. Hypotension caused by blood loss

V. TRUE OR FALSE

Indicate whether each statement is True (T) or False (F).

_____ 1. Adrenergic nerve fibers have only alpha- or beta-receptors.

_____ 2. Adrenergic drugs may bind to alpha-, beta-, or alpha/beta-receptor sites.

VI. MULTIPLE CHOICE

Circle the letter of the best answer.

1. _____ mimic the activity of the sympathetic nervous system.
   a. Cholinergic drugs
   b. Adrenergic drugs
   c. Cholinergic blocking drugs
   d. Adrenergic blocking drugs
   e. None of the above

2. A neurotransmitter is
   a. a chemical substance released at nerve endings to help transient nerve impulses.
   b. a drug that raises the blood pressure because it constricts the blood vessels.
   c. a specific protein-like macromolecule required for a drug's action at the cellular level.
   d. a branch of the autonomic nervous system.

3. Adrenergic drugs generally produce which of the following responses?
   a. Increased heart rate
   b. Increased use of glucose
   c. Wakefulness
   d. Relaxation of smooth muscles of the bronchi
   e. All of the above

4. Adrenergic drugs can be used to treat shock because they _____.
   a. decrease cardiac output and cause vasodilation
   b. improve myocardial contractility and cause vasoconstriction
   c. allow hypotension to occur
   d. cause bradycardia
   e. can keep the kidneys, brain, and heart alive

5. All of the following, except one, is a common adverse reaction of adrenergic drugs. Indicate the exception.
   a. Cardiac arrhythmias
   b. Headache
   c. Insomnia
   d. Drowsiness
   e. Increased blood pressure

6. Which of the following is a part of the central nervous system?
   a. The parasympathetic nervous system
   b. The sympathetic nervous system
   c. The brain
   d. The spinal cord
   e. Both c and d

7. The somatic nervous system is the branch that
   a. controls the sensation and voluntary movement.
   b. regulates the expenditure of energy and has key effects in stressful situations.
   c. is partly responsible for activities such as slowing the heart rate, digesting the food, and eliminating the body wastes.
   d. controls the function essential for survival.

8. Acetylcholine is
   a. a neurotransmitter that inactivates acetylcholine.
   b. a neurotransmitter in the parasympathetic nervous system.
   c. an adrenergic drug.
   d. a receptor site.

9. The drug _____ is used to treat orthostatic hypotension.
   a. epinephrine
   b. isoproterenol
   c. norepinephrine
   d. midodrine

10. Levophed is the trade name for
    a. midodrine.
    b. dopamine.
    c. dobutamine.
    d. norepinephrine.

11. A contraindication for dopamine is:
    a. ventricular fibrillation.
    b. narrow-angle glaucoma.
    c. severe organic heart disease.
    d. acute renal disease.

12. A patient with pheochromocytoma should not be given
    a. epinephrine.
    b. norepinephrine.
    c. isoproterenol.
    d. dopamine.

13. When epinephrine is administered with a _____, the patient has an increased risk of sympathomimetic effects.
    a. tricyclic antidepressant
    b. beta blocker
    c. antihistamine
    d. antianginal

14. All of the following are clinical manifestations of shock except
    a. acidosis.
    b. urinary output <100 ml/hour.
    c. pallor and cyanosis.
    d. hypotension.

15. Precautions when giving midodrine include
    a. checking the blood pressure before initiating therapy in the lying and sitting position.
    b. giving the drug only when the patient is out of bed.
    c. monitoring the heart rate and the blood pressure frequently.
    d. All of the above

VII. RECALL FACTS

Indicate whether the listed adrenergic drug is an alpha (A), a beta (B), or an alpha/beta (AB) drug.

ABOUT ADRENERGIC DRUGS

____ 1. Phenylephrine

____ 2. Isoproterenol

____ 3. Epinephrine

Indicate which of the following statements are facts with an F. If the statement is not a fact, leave the line blank.

ABOUT MANAGING THE PATIENT IN SHOCK

____ 1. When an adrenergic drug is to be given for shock, the patient's blood pressure, pulse rate and quality, and respiratory rate and rhythm are first assessed.

____ 2. The initial pharmacologic intervention is aimed at supporting urinary output.

____ 3. Some hypotensive episodes require the use of a less potent vasopressor, such as norepinephrine.

____ 4. The patient's heart rate, blood pressure, and ECG are monitored continuously.

____ 5. Management of shock is aimed at providing basic life support while attempting to correct the underlying cause.

VIII. FILL IN THE BLANKS

Fill in the blanks using words from the list below.

cardiac glycoside	contraction	monoamine oxidase inhibitor	epinephrine	constriction
midodrine	narrow angle glaucoma	coronary insufficiency	hypovolemic shock	neurogenic shock

1. Supine hypertension is a potentially dangerous adverse reaction of _____ .

2. _____ is a contraindication for giving epinephrine.

3. Adrenergic drugs are used cautiously for patients with _____ .

4. For patients with Parkinson disease, _____ is used with caution.

5. The effects of dopamine may be increased when given a(n) _____ .

6. When midodrine is given with a(n) _____ , arrhythmias can occur.

7. The sympathetic effect on the blood vessels is _____ .

8. The adrenergic effect on the radial muscle of the iris is _____ .

9. _____ occurs when the extracellular fluid volume is significantly diminished.

10. _____ occurs as a result of blockade of neurohumoral outflow.

IX. LIST

List the requested number of items.

1. List four conditions that adrenergic drugs may be used to treat.

    a. _____

    b. _____

    c. _____

    d. _____

2. List the five types of shock.

    a. _____

    b. _____

    c. _____

    d. _____

    e. _____

3. List four responses of the central nervous system to adrenergic drugs.

    a. _____

    b. _____

    c. _____

    d. _____

4. List five responses of the sympathetic nervous system to adrenergic drugs.

    a. _____

    b. _____

    c. _____

    d. _____

    e. _____

5. List the four uses of isoproterenol.

    a. _____

    b. _____

    c. _____

    d. _____

6. List the five clinical manifestations of shock.

    a. _____

    b. _____

    c. _____

    d. _____

    e. _____

7. List the three organs that are compromised by shock.

    a. _____

    b. _____

    c. _____

8. List the four contraindications to giving midodrine.

    a. _____

    b. _____

    c. _____

    d. _____

9. List five conditions for which adrenergic drugs are given with caution.

    a. _____

    b. _____

    c. _____

    d. _____

    e. _____

10. List four techniques that help manage the anorexia caused by adrenergic drugs.

    a. _____

    b. _____

    c. _____

    d. _____

X. CLINICAL APPLICATIONS

1. Mr. S. is in cardiogenic shock. What drugs do you
   anticipate might be given to treat this?

XI. CASE STUDY

Mr. L. is having difficulty sleeping since being put on an
adrenergic medication.

1. One intervention to help in his care would be to
   a. awaken him to take his blood pressure every
      2 hours.
   b. avoid disturbance of his sleep.
   c. promote an exercise routine before bedtime.
   d. offer iced drinks at bedtime.

2. Which of the following drinks would be discour-
   aged after the late afternoon?
   a. Warm milk
   b. Cold milk
   c. Coffee
   d. Caffeine free beverage

3. Which of the following approaches would be used
   for food intake?
   a. Bedtime snack
   b. Three large meals a day
   c. A large meal before bed
   d. Hold breakfast

12

Adrenergic Blocking Drugs

I. MATCH THE FOLLOWING

Match the generic adrenergic blocking drug from Column A with the trade name of the drug from Column B.

COLUMN A

____ 1. phentolamine

____ 2. betaxolol

____ 3. propranolol

____ 4. esmolol

____ 5. labetalol

____ 6. clonidine

____ 7. carvedilol

COLUMN B

A. Brevibloc

B. Regitine

C. Kerlone

D. Normodyne

E. Catapres

F. Coreg

G. Inderal

II. MATCH THE FOLLOWING

Match the adrenergic blocking drug from Column A with the corresponding contraindication from Column B.

COLUMN A

____ 1. Alpha-adrenergic blocking drugs

____ 2. Beta-adrenergic blocking drugs

____ 3. Antiadrenergic blocking drugs (centrally acting)

____ 4. Antiadrenergic blocking drugs (peripherally acting)

COLUMN B

A. Sinus bradycardia, asthma

B. Active hepatic disease

C. Coronary artery disease

D. Renal impairment, congestive heart failure

III. TRUE OR FALSE

Indicate whether each statement is True (T) or False (F).

____ 1. Beta-adrenergic blocking drugs work to stimulate receptors in the heart and cause the heart rate to increase.

____ 2. Beta-adrenergic blocking drugs can result in a greater risk of adverse reactions for older adults.

____ 3. Centrally acting antiadrenergic drugs have a different action than peripherally acting anti-

adrenergic drugs, but both produce the same basic results.

____ 4. Adverse reactions of peripherally acting antiadrenergic drugs include dry mouth, drowsiness, anorexia, and weakness.

____ 5. Peripheral vasodilation is the result of administering an alpha/beta-adrenergic blocking drug.

IV. MULTIPLE CHOICE

Circle the letter of the best answer.

1. The first dose effect is
   a. a feeling of light-headedness and hypotension with the first dose of a drug.
   b. an unusually strong therapeutic effect experienced by some patients with the first dose of a medication.
   c. an unusually weak therapeutic effect experienced by some patients with the first dose of a medication.
   d. Both a and b

2. Postural hypotension
   a. is also known as orthostatic hypotension.
   b. is a feeling of light-headedness and dizziness.
   c. occurs after a sudden position change.
   d. All of the above

3. Measures to minimize the adverse reactions from adrenergic blocking drugs include all of the following except?
   a. Have the patient sit on the side of the bed for 1 minute before standing
   b. Instruct the patient to rise slowly from a sitting position or lying position
   c. Stay with the patient while they are standing in one place and when walking
   d. Encourage the patient to take hot showers and baths

4. Halothane increases the effects of
   a. labetalol.
   b. clonidine.
   c. digoxin.
   d. carvedilol.

5. Adverse reactions of labetalol include
   a. fatigue.
   b. drowsiness.
   c. insomnia.
   d. weakness.
   e. All of the above

6. Alpha-adrenergic blocking drugs _____.
   a. stimulate vasodilation
   b. can be used to treat hypertension from pheochromocytoma
   c. may have adverse reactions of weakness, orthostatic hypotension, or cardiac arrhythmias
   d. are contraindicated in patients with coronary artery disease
   e. All of the above

7. In which of the following conditions are beta-adrenergic blocking drugs used for treatment?
   a. Hypertension
   b. Congestive heart failure
   c. Glaucoma
   d. Cardiac arrhythmias
   e. Answers a, c, and d

8. Patients in whom beta-adrenergic drugs are contraindicated are those _____.
   a. with a known hypersensitivity to the drugs
   b. with sinus bradycardia
   c. with heart failure
   d. with asthma or emphysema
   e. All of the above

9. Which patient should not be prescribed an alpha/beta-adrenergic blocking drug?
   a. A patient with diarrhea
   b. A patient with bronchial asthma
   c. A patient with myocardial infarction
   d. A patient with a gastrointestinal disorder
   e. A patient with hypotension

10. Adverse reactions of carvedilol include
    a. fatigue.
    b. hypertension.
    c. cardiac insufficiency.
    d. Both a and c

11. Alpha/beta-adrenergic blocking drugs are used with caution in patients with
    a. drug-controlled congestive heart failure.
    b. chronic bronchitis.
    c. impaired hepatic or cardiac function.
    d. diabetes.
    e. All of the above

12. Glaucoma
    a. is a narrowing or blockage of the drainage channels between the anterior and posterior chambers of the eye.
    b. results in decreased intraocular pressure in the eye.
    c. may cause blindness if it is left untreated.
    d. Both a and c

13. Drugs used to treat glaucoma include
    a. nadolol.
    b. betaxolol.
    c. timolol.
    d. Both b and c
    e. Both a and b

14. The effects of beta-blockers may be decreased when used with
    a. indomethacin.
    b. ibuprofen.
    c. sulindac.
    d. barbiturates.
    e. All of the above

V. RECALL FACTS

Indicate which of the following statements are facts with an F. If the statement is not a fact, leave the line blank.

ABOUT BETA-ADRENERGIC BLOCKING DRUGS

____ 1. They are used primarily in the treatment of hypertension

____ 2. Some of these drugs have additional uses, such as the use of propranolol for migraine headaches and nadolol for angina pectoris

____ 3. They can be used topically as eye drops

____ 4. May be used to prevent another heart attack in patients with a recent myocardial nfarction

____ 5. They are used in the treatment of certain cardiac arrhythmias

____ 6. They are used to slow the progression of congestive heart failure

____ 7. They are used to treat pheochromocytoma

Indicate whether the listed adrenergic blocking drug is an alpha (A), a beta (B), or an alpha/beta (AB) drug.

ABOUT ADRENERGIC BLOCKING DRUGS

____ 1. carvedilol

____ 2. betaxolol

____ 3. phentolamine

____ 4. timolol

____ 5. propanolol

____ 6. labetalol

VI. FILL IN THE BLANKS

Fill in the blanks using words from the list below.

glaucoma	anorexia	reserpine	adrenergic blocking drug	first dose effect
propranolol	congestive heart failure	diuretics	terazosin	

1. _____ is a narrowing or blockage of the drainage channels of the eye.

2. A serious adverse reaction of beta-adrenergic blocking drugs includes the symptoms of _____ .

3. A(n) _____ is generally self-limiting and in most cases does not recur after the initial period of therapy.

4. _____ is an adverse reaction on centrally acting antiadrenergic drugs.

5. A common adverse reaction of a(n) _____ is postural hypotension.

6. _____ is contraindicated in patients with active peptic ulcer or ulcerative colitis or depression.

7. Food may affect the absorption of
   _____.

8. _____ may increase the hypoten-
   sive effects of beta-adrenergic blocking drugs.

9. _____ may be used in patients
   with benign prostatic hyperplasia.

VII. LIST

List the requested number of items.

1. List the three uses of phentolamine.

   a. _____

   b. _____

   c. _____

2. List the five effects of alpha-adrenergic blocking
   drugs.

   a. _____

   b. _____

   c. _____

   d. _____

   e. _____

3. List the four groups of adrenergic blocking drugs.

   a. _____

   b. _____

   c. _____

   d. _____

4. List four examples of beta-adrenergic blocking
   drugs.

   a. _____

   b. _____

   c. _____

   d. _____

5. List four things that a health care worker could do
   to help a patient minimize the adverse reaction of
   hypotension.

   a. _____

   b. _____

   c. _____

   d. _____

6. List four uses of beta-adrenergic blocking drugs.

   a. _____

   b. _____

   c. _____

   d. _____

7. List four symptoms that older patients on beta-
   adrenergic blocking drugs should be monitored for.

   a. _____

   b. _____

   c. _____

   d. _____

8. List five situations in which beta-adrenergic
   blocking drugs are contraindicated.

   a. _____

   b. _____

   c. _____

   d. _____

   e. _____

9. List three types of patients for whom beta-adrenergic
   drugs are given with caution.

   a. _____

   b. _____

   c. _____

10. List the three actions of antiadrenergic drugs.

    a. _____

    b. _____

    c. _____

VIII. CLINICAL APPLICATIONS

1. Your father has been diagnosed with hypertension and must monitor his blood pressure daily at home. What could you suggest to your father to help ensure that he gets an accurate blood pressure reading?

IX. CASE STUDY

Mr. J. was put on the beta-adrenergic blocking drug timolol for his glaucoma. The medical staff has instructed Mr. J. about the pathophysiology of glaucoma.

1. Elements of pathophysiology include
   a. glaucoma is a narrowing or blockage of the drainage channels of the eye.
   b. glaucoma results in increased intraocular pressure in the eye.
   c. blindness, it may occur if glaucoma is left untreated.
   d. All of the above

2. Education about instillation of Mr. J.'s eye medication should include
   a. a demonstration of how to use eye drops correctly.
   b. the importance of staying on the eye drop instillation schedule.
   c. the fact that delay or discontinuance of the drug may result in a marked increase in intraocular pressure which could lead to blindness.
   d. contacting the health care provider if eye pain, excessive tearing, or any change in vision occur.
   e. All of the above

13

Cholinergic Drugs

I. MATCH THE FOLLOWING

Match the generic cholinergic drug from Column A with the corresponding trade name from Column B.

COLUMN A	COLUMN B
____ 1. ambenonium	A. Duvoid
____ 2. pyridostigmine bromide	B. Isopto Carpine
____ 3. bethanechol chloride	C. Mytelase
____ 4. neostigmine	D. Mestinon
____ 5. pilocarpine	E. Prostigmin
____ 6. edrophonium	F. Tensilon
____ 7. carbachol	G. Isopto Carbachol

II. MATCH THE FOLLOWING

Match the term from Column A with the correct definition from Column B.

COLUMN A

____ 1. Myasthenia gravis

____ 2. Cholinergic crisis

____ 3. Cholinergic drugs

____ 4. Urinary retention

____ 5. Glaucoma

____ 6. Myopia

____ 7. Visual acuity

COLUMN B

A. A disease that causes fatigue of skeletal muscles because of the lack of acetylcholine released at the nerve endings of parasympathetic nerve fibers

B. Sharpness of vision

C. Disorder of increased pressure within the eye

D. Cholinergic drug toxicity

E. Nearsightedness

F. Condition where urination is impaired

G. Drugs that mimic the activity of the parasympathetic nervous system

III. TRUE OR FALSE

Indicate whether each statement is True (T) or False (F).

____ 1. A direct-acting cholinergic drug acts like the neurohormone acetylcholine.

____ 2. Cholinergic drugs, with the exception of topical administration, are selective and specific receptor-dependent in their actions.

IV. MULTIPLE CHOICE

Circle the letter of the best answer.

1. Cholinergic drugs may
   a. act like the neurohormone ACh.
   b. inhibit the release of the neurohormone AChE.
   c. be called direct-acting cholinergics.
   d. may be called indirect-acting cholinergics.
   e. All of the above

2. The neurohormone AChE
   a. shortens the active period of the ACh produced naturally by the body.
   b. prolongs the activity of ACh.
   c. inhibits the release of ACh.
   d. None of the above

3. Myasthenia gravis is
   a. a disease that causes fatigue of the skeletal muscles.
   b. caused by the lack of acetylcholine released at the nerve endings of parasympathetic fibers.
   c. caused by administration of beta-adrenergic blocking drugs.
   d. Both a and b

4. Mytelase is the trade name for
   a. bethanechol.
   b. carbachol.
   c. ambenonium.
   d. edrophonium.

5. _____ is the drug used to help make the diagnosis of myasthenia gravis.
   a. Edrophonium
   b. Neostigmine
   c. Pilocarpine hydrochloride
   d. Pyridostigmine bromide

6. An adverse reaction to pyridostigmine may include
   a. temporary reduction in visual acuity.
   b. cardiac arrhythmias.
   c. bowel cramps.
   d. urgency.

7. Key points related to instilling eye medication include which of the following?
   a. Keep the bottle tightly closed
   b. Do not wash the tip of the dropper
   c. Do not put the dropper down on a table or other surface
   d. Do not let the tip of the dropper touch the eye
   e. All of the above

8. Information given to the glaucoma patient who is prescribed a cholinergic drug includes which of the following?
   a. Eye drops may sting when put in the eye; this is normal but usually temporary
   b. Be cautious while driving or performing any task that requires visual acuity
   c. Local irritation and headache may occur at the beginning of the therapy
   d. Notify the health care provider if you have abdominal cramping, diarrhea, or excessive salivation
   e. All of the above

9. Patients with myasthenia gravis and their families should be instructed to
   a. keep a record of response to the drug therapy.
   b. bring the response record to each clinic visit.
   c. wear or carry identification indicating that they have myasthenia gravis.
   d. keep a written or printed description of the signs and symptoms of drug over- and under-dose.
   e. All of the above

10. Bethanechol is used for
    a. myasthenia gravis.
    b. bowel cramps.
    c. urinary retention.
    d. glaucoma.

11. Cholinergic drugs are commonly used to treat patients with _____.
    a. myocardial infarction
    b. glaucoma
    c. myasthenia gravis
    d. urinary retention
    e. Answers b, c, and d

12. Which of the following cholinergic drugs might be prescribed for a patient with myasthenia gravis?
    a. Pilocarpine
    b. Ambenonium
    c. Pyridostigmine
    d. Bethanechol chloride
    e. Either b or c

13. A patient in a cholinergic crisis may exhibit all *except* which of the following symptoms?
    a. Severe abdominal cramping
    b. Clenching of the jaw
    c. Migraine headache
    d. Excessive salivation
    e. Diarrhea

14. A patient receiving a cholinergic drug for treatment of myasthenia gravis _____.
    a. may need to adjust their drug dosage according to their needs
    b. must be observed for symptoms of drug overdose
    c. must be observed for symptoms of drug underdose
    d. All of the above

V. RECALL FACTS

Indicate which of the following statements are facts with an F. If the statement is not a fact, leave the line blank.

ABOUT MYASTHENIA GRAVIS

____ 1. Neostigmine is a drug used for treatment

____ 2. Edrophonium is used to help establish the diagnosis

____ 3. Bethanechol is used in difficult cases

____ 4. The disease causes increased strength in the skeletal muscles

____ 5. It is characterized by a lack of ACh release at the nerve endings of the parasympathetic nerve fibers

____ 6. Drug dosage adjustments may be frequent

Indicate whether the listed cholinergic drugs are used for myasthenia gravis (MG), urinary retention (UR), glaucoma (G), or more than one disorder.

ABOUT CHOLINERGIC DRUGS

____ 1. ambenonium

____ 2. bethanechol chloride

____ 3. carbachol topical

____ 4. neostigmine

____ 5. pilocarpine HCl

____ 6. pyridostigmine bromide

VI. FILL IN THE BLANKS

Fill in the blanks using words from the list below.

5–10 minutes	indirect-acting cholinergics	atropine	miosis
urinary retention	clenching of the jaw	drug-induced myopia	direct-acting cholinergics
neurohormone	drooping of the eyelids		

1. _____ is one of the symptoms of cholinergic crisis.

2. _____ is a sign of drug underdosage in myasthenia gravis.

3. Patients with _____ must be monitored for fluid intake and output.

4. The anti-cholinergic drug, _____, is used as an antidote to cholinergic drug overdose.

5. Use of cholinergic eyedrops may cause _____.

6. _____ is constriction of the iris.

7. A patient being treated with a cholinergic drug for urinary retention can expect urination to occur within _____ of subcutaneous drug administration.

8. _____ are drugs that act like Ach.

9. Ach is a _____.

10. _____ are drugs that inhibit the release of AChE.

VII. LIST

List the requested number of items.

1. List the three conditions for which cholinergic drugs may be prescribed.

   a. _____

   b. _____

   c. _____

2. List three signs of underdosage of cholinergic drugs.

   a. _____

   b. _____

   c. _____

3. List four signs of overdosage of cholinergic drugs.

   a. _____

   b. _____

   c. _____

   d. _____

4. List four important care aspects for the patient with urinary retention who has been given a cholinergic drug.

   a. _____

   b. _____

   c. _____

   d. _____

5. List five symptoms of cholinergic toxicity or cholinergic crisis.

   a. _____

   b. _____

   c. _____

   d. _____

   e. _____

6. List four adverse reactions to ambenonium.

   a. _____

   b. _____

   c. _____

   d. _____

7. List five adverse reactions to neostigmine.

   a. _____

   b. _____

   c. _____

   d. _____

   e. _____

8. List four common adverse effects of cholinergic drugs.

   a. _____

   b. _____

   c. _____

   d. _____

9. List four important aspects of administering a cholinergic drug to a glaucoma patient.

   a. _____

   b. _____

   c. _____

   d. _____

10. List the three drugs that can be used to treat myasthenia gravis.

    a. _____

    b. _____

    c. _____

VIII. CLINICAL APPLICATIONS

1. Mr. J. has been diagnosed with myasthenia gravis. He and his family are eager to learn more about the disease and what they must do. What information is important for them to know about his care? What possible drugs may be prescribed to him?

IX. CASE STUDY

Mr. W. has been having difficulty with urinary retention. His doctor has ordered a dose of bethanechol subcutaneously for Mr. W.

1. What should you anticipate related to his care?

   a. The drug will start to act after he returns home
   b. Urination usually occurs 5–15 minutes after subcutaneous administration.
   c. Urination usually occurs 30–90 minutes after subcutaneous administration.
   d. None of the above

2. Mr. W.'s condition requires that certain aspects of care are carried out while he is in the hospital. These may include which of the following?

   a. Monitoring for the fluid intake and output
   b. Monitoring for the response to medications
   c. Ensuring the call light is within reach
   d. Ensuring a urinal or a bedpan is in easy reach
   e. All the above

3. Other drugs that might be used for Mr. W. would include

   a. neostigmine.
   b. carbachol.
   c. edrophonium.
   d. pilocarpine.

14

Cholinergic Blocking Drugs (Anticholinergics)

I. MATCH THE FOLLOWING

Match the generic cholinergic blocking drug from Column A with the corresponding trade name from Column B.

COLUMN A

____ 1. flavoxate

____ 2. trihexyphenidyl

____ 3. glycopyrrolate

____ 4. dicyclomine HCL

____ 5. methscopolamine

____ 6. l-hyoscyamine sulfate

____ 7. mepenzolate bromide

____ 8. propantheline bromide

COLUMN B

A. Urispas

B. Pamine

C. Robinul

D. Bentyl

E. Artane

F. Pro-banthine

G. Cantil

H. Anaspaz

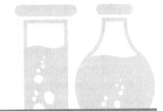

II. MATCH THE FOLLOWING

Match the term from Column A with the correct term from Column B.

COLUMN A

____ 1. Cholinergic blocking drugs

____ 2. Acetylcholine

____ 3. Parasympathomimetic blocking drugs

____ 4. Parkinsonism

____ 5. A cholinergic effect

____ 6. Cantil

____ 7. Flavoxate

____ 8. Artane

COLUMN B

A. Another name for cholinergic blocking drugs

B. Dryness of the mouth

C. Drugs that impede certain parasympathetic nervous system functions

D. Used as adjunctive treatment for peptic ulcer

E. Neurotransmitter blocked by cholinergic blocking drugs

F. A condition for which atropine may be used

G. Used for extrapyramidal effects of parkinsonism

H. Used for dysuria

III. TRUE OR FALSE

Indicate whether each statement is True (T) or False (F).

____ 1. Cholinergic blocking drugs have a variety of uses because of their widespread effects on many organs and structures.

IV. MULTIPLE CHOICE

Circle the letter of the best answer.

1. Cholinergic blocking drugs may be called
   a. anticholinergics.
   b. parasympathomimetic blocking drugs.
   c. sympathetic blocking drugs.
   d. Both a and b

2. _____ block the action of the neurotransmitter acetylcholine in the parasympathetic nervous system.
   a. Cholinergic drugs
   b. Adrenergic drugs
   c. Adrenergic blocking drugs
   d. Cholinergic blocking drugs
   e. None of the above

3. When the activity of acetylcholine is inhibited,
   a. nerve impulses along the parasympathetic nerves travel more easily.
   b. nerve impulses traveling along parasympathetic nerve fibers cannot pass to the effector organ or the structure.
   c. there is an increased activity in the sympathetic nervous system.
   d. None of the above

4. An idiosyncratic reaction to a drug is
   a. an expected effect.
   b. an unexpected effect.
   c. an unusual drug effect.
   d. a latent drug effect.
   e. Both b and c

5. An idiosyncratic effect of scopolamine may include
   a. excitement.
   b. delirium.
   c. restlessness.
   d. All of the above

6. Cholinergic blocking drugs may produce which of the following responses in the central nervous system?
   a. Dreamless sleep
   b. Wakefulness
   c. Drowsiness
   d. Mild stimulation
   e. Answers a, c, and d

7. Cholinergic blocking drugs may produce which of the following responses in the urinary tract?
   a. Increase in the pulse rate
   b. Dilatation of smooth muscles in the ureters
   c. Dilatation of smooth muscles in the kidney pelvis
   d. Contraction of the detrusor muscle of the bladder
   e. Answers b, c, and d

8. Atropine is used for all of the following except
   a. pylorospasm.
   b. reduction of bronchial and oral secretions.
   c. tachycardia.
   d. ureteral and biliary colic.

9. Side effects of atropine include which of the following?
   a. Drowsiness
   b. Blurred vision
   c. Tachycardia
   d. Dry mouth
   e. All of the above

10. The effects of cholinergic blocking drugs on the respiratory tract include
    a. drying of the secretions of the mouth and the nose.
    b. relaxation of smooth muscles of the bronchi.
    c. slight bronchodilatation.
    d. drying of the secretions of the throat and the bronchi.
    e. All of the above

11. Uses of the drug Robinul include all of the following except
    a. peptic ulcer.
    b. to terminate tachycardia.
    c. to reduce the bronchial and oral secretions with anesthesia.
    d. to protect against the peripheral muscarinic effects of cholinergic agents.

12. Which of the following may be recommended to a patient who has been put on a cholinergic blocking drug, to help prevent the often accompanying constipation?
    a. Increase fluid intake up to 2,000 ml daily (if health permits)
    b. Eat a diet high in fiber
    c. Get adequate exercise
    d. Chloride prescription for a stool softener
    e. All of the above

13. Patients who are experiencing photophobia while on a cholinergic drug, which of the following may be recommended?

    a. Wear sunglasses when outside
    b. Keep rooms dimly lit
    c. Close curtains and blinds to eliminate bright sunlight in the room
    d. Schedule outdoor activities before taking the first dose of the drug in the morning if possible
    e. All of the above

14. Side effects of cholinergic blocking drugs include all of the following except

    a. drowsiness.
    b. dysphagia.
    c. dizziness.
    d. blurred vision.

15. Care issues and cautions for patients receiving a cholinergic blocking agent as a preoperative medication include

    a. urinating before the preoperative medication is given.
    b. drowsiness and extreme dryness of the mouth and the nose will occur approximately 20–30 minutes after the drug is given.
    c. staying in bed with the side rails raised after the drug is administered.
    d. All of the above.

V. RECALL FACTS

Indicate which of the following statements are facts with an F. If the statement is not a fact, leave the line blank.

ABOUT MANAGING ADVERSE REACTIONS OF CHOLINERGIC BLOCKING AGENTS

_____ 1. Heat prostration may be a problem for elderly or debilitated patients in hot weather.

_____ 2. Elderly patients receiving a cholinergic blocking drug should be observed closely for signs of mental confusion, agitation, or other adverse reactions.

_____ 3. Photophobia and blurred vision are rarely a concern for patients on cholinergic blocking agents.

_____ 4. Mouth dryness will go away after the cholinergic blocking drug is used for awhile.

_____ 5. Objects that may obstruct walking should be moved out of the patients' way.

_____ 6. Patients experiencing constipation, who are not fluid restricted, may increase their fluid intake up to 2,000 ml per day.

Indicate which cholinergic blocking drugs are used for the urinary tract (U), the gastrointestinal tract (G), Parkinsonism (P), or the respiratory tract (R). Some drugs may have multiple answers.

ABOUT CHOLINERGIC BLOCKING DRUGS

_____ 1. Atropine

_____ 2. Dicyclomine HCl

_____ 3. Flavoxate

_____ 4. Glycopyrrolate

_____ 5. Mepenzolate

_____ 6. Methscopolamine

_____ 7. Propantheline bromide

_____ 8. Trihexyphenidyl

VI. FILL IN THE BLANKS

Fill in the blanks using words from the list below.

glaucoma   drowsiness   cholinergic blocking drug   acetylcholine   scopolamine
drug idiosyncrasy   atropine   mydriasis   cycloplegia   Artane

1. _____ is an adverse effect of cholinergic blocking drugs.

2. _____ is a neurotransmitter.

3. _____ occasionally causes excitement, delirium, and restlessness.

4. A(n) _____ is an unexpected or
   unusual drug effect.

5. A common adverse reaction of a(n)
   _____ is dryness of the mouth.

6. Cholinergic blocking drugs are contraindicated in
   patients with _____.

7. A drug used to treat pylorospasm is
   _____.

8. _____ is used to treat the extrapyramidal effects caused by antipsychotic drugs.

9. Paralysis of accommodation or inability to focus
   the eye is _____.

10. One of the adverse effects of anticholinergic drugs
    on the eyes is _____.

VII. LIST

List the requested number of items.

1. List four drugs used to treat peptic ulcer.

   a. _____

   b. _____

   c. _____

   d. _____

2. List three responses of the central nervous system
   to cholinergic blocking drugs.

   a. _____

   b. _____

   c. _____

3. List three responses of the gastrointestinal tract to
   cholinergic blocking drugs.

   a. _____

   b. _____

   c. _____

4. List three drugs used for treating ureteral colic,
   dysuria, or prostatitis.

   a. _____

   b. _____

   c. _____

5. List four measures that would prevent heat
   prostration.

   a. _____

   b. _____

   c. _____

   d. _____

6. List three measures that would help prevent
   constipation.

   a. _____

   b. _____

   c. _____

7. List four precautions to tell family members of the elderly patient on a cholinergic blocking drug.

   a. _____

   b. _____

   c. _____

   d. _____

8. List the five of the most common "anticholinergic effects" or adverse effects of cholinergic blocking drugs.

   a. _____

   b. _____

   c. _____

   d. _____

   e. _____

9. List four responses of the respiratory tract to cholinergic blocking drugs.

   a. _____

   b. _____

   c. _____

   d. _____

10. List four adverse reactions to the drug trihexyphenidyl (Artane).

   a. _____

   b. _____

   c. _____

   d. _____

VIII. CLINICAL APPLICATIONS

1. Mrs. P's health care provider has prescribed, Pamine, a cholinergic blocking drug for the treatment of her peptic ulcer. Knowing that a dry mouth is a common adverse reaction of this medication, the health care provider asks you to give Mrs. P some helpful hints for dealing with the potential problem. What might you suggest to Mrs. P to help her?

IX. CASE STUDY

Mrs. C., age 79, has been diagnosed with a peptic ulcer at her last checkup. Her physician has ordered a medication for her to take and she and her family have been given special instructions related to her care.

1. What medication was Mrs. C. most likely prescribed?
   a. Flavoxate
   b. Dicyclomine HCl
   c. Glycopyrrolate
   d. Atropine

2. What specific instructions were given about the timing of her drug dosage?
   a. The drug should be taken exactly as prescribed.
   b. The medication most likely would be taken 30 minutes before meals or between meals.
   c. The medication would be taken with food.
   d. Both a and b

3. Mrs. C. likes to garden and is concerned about heat prostration while on her medication. What advice should she be given related to this?
   a. Avoid going outside on hot, sunny days.
   b. Use fans to stay cool if the day is extremely warm.
   c. Sponge the skin with cool water if other cooling measures are not available.
   d. Wear loose-fitting clothes in warm weather.
   e. All of the above

DRUGS THAT AFFECT THE RESPIRATORY SYSTEM

15

Bronchodilators and Antiasthma Drugs

I. MATCH THE FOLLOWING

Match the term from Column A with the correct definition from Column B.

COLUMN A

_____ 1. Sympathomimetics

_____ 2. Theophyllinization

_____ 3. Leukotrienes

_____ 4. Xanthine derivatives

_____ 5. Emphysema

_____ 6. Chronic bronchitis

_____ 7. Dyspnea

_____ 8. Chronic obstructive pulmonary disease

COLUMN B

A. Substances that are released by the body during the inflammatory process and constrict the bronchia

B. A lung disorder in which the terminal bronchioles or the alveoli become enlarged and plugged with mucus

C. Difficulty breathing

D. Drugs that mimic the activities of the sympathetic nervous system

E. Name given collectively to emphysema and chronic bronchitis

F. Abnormal inflammation and possible infection of the bronchi

G. Process of giving the patient a higher initial dose of theophylline to bring the drug levels of theophylline to a therapeutic range more quickly

H. Drugs that stimulate the central nervous system and result in bronchodilation

II. MATCH THE FOLLOWING

Match the generic corticosteroid, leukotriene, or mast cell stabilizer from Column A with the correct trade name from Column B.

COLUMN A   COLUMN B

____ 1. budesonide   A. Pulmicort

____ 2. flunisolide   B. Flovent

____ 3. beclomethasone dipropionate   C. Singulair

____ 4. ciclesonide   D. Zyflo

____ 5. cromolyn   E. AeroBid

____ 6. fluticasone propionate   F. Beconase AQ

____ 7. zileuton   G. Alvesco

____ 8. zafirlukast   H. Accolate

____ 9. montelukast sodium   I. Nasalcrom

____ 10. mometasone   J. Asmanex

III. MATCH THE FOLLOWING

Match the drug from Column A with the correct classification from Column B. You may use an answer more than once.

COLUMN A   COLUMN B

____ 1. albuterol sulfate   A. Xanthine derivative

____ 2. epinephrine   B. Sympathomimetic

____ 3. theophylline

____ 4. dyphylline

____ 5. metaproterenol sulfate

____ 6. salmeterol

____ 7. aminophylline

____ 8. terbutaline

____ 9. ephedrine sulfate

____ 10. arformoterol

____ 11. salmeterol

____ 12. pirbuterol acetate

IV. TRUE OR FALSE

Indicate whether each statement is True (T) or False (F).

____ 1. Asthma is an irreversible obstructive disease of the lower airway.

____ 2. Excessive use of an inhaled sympathomimetic bronchodilator can result in paradoxical bronchospasm.

____ 3. Additive adrenergic effects can occur when two sympathomimetic drugs are used concurrently.

____ 4. Xanthine derivatives stimulate the central nervous system, resulting in bronchodilation caused by relaxation of the smooth muscles in the bronchi.

____ 5. Inhalation is the route of administration most often used for corticosteroids.

____ 6. Vertigo, headaches, and oral fungal infections are adverse reactions of inhaled corticosteroids.

____ 7. Montelukast works by stimulating leukotriene receptor sites in the respiratory tract.

____ 8. Leukotriene receptor antagonists and leukotriene formation inhibitors are the drugs of choice during an acute asthma attack.

____ 9. Zileuton therapy management includes regular monitoring of the patient's ALT levels.

____ 10. Zileuton is contraindicated in patients with active liver disease.

____ 11. Mast cell stabilizers act by inhibiting mast cells from releasing substances that stimulate inflammation and bronchoconstriction.

____ 12. Mast cell stabilizers are contraindicated in patients during an acute asthma attack.

V. MULTIPLE CHOICE

Circle the letter of the best answer.

1. Allergic asthma _____.
   a. causes the release of histamine
   b. causes carbon dioxide to be trapped in the alveoli
   c. causes the production of immunoglobulin E
   d. can be triggered by an allergen
   e. All of the above

2. Bronchodilators are drugs that are used to relieve bronchospasm caused by _____.
   a. emphysema
   b. bronchial pneumonia
   c. chronic bronchitis
   d. bronchial asthma
   e. Answers a, c, and d

3. The nervousness, anxiety, and restlessness observed in patients who are being treated for difficulty breathing with a sympathomimetic may be caused by _____.
   a. environmental factors
   b. the respiratory disorder itself
   c. an adverse drug reaction
   d. Both b and c
   e. Answers a, b, and c

4. Salmeterol is contraindicated in _____.
   a. patients with depression
   b. acute bronchospasm
   c. congestive heart failure
   d. renal failure
   e. None of the above

5. Theophyllinization _____.
   a. is used for acute respiratory situations
   b. uses xanthine derivatives
   c. involves giving the patient a loading dose of theophylline
   d. Both a and c
   e. Answers a, b, and c

6. Mrs. A has been taking theophylline for her respiratory disorder. As the health care worker assigned to her, what might you tell Mrs. A to help her minimize possible adverse reactions from this medication?
   a. Lay in a prone position
   b. Remain upright and sleep with the head of the bed elevated
   c. Walking increases the effectiveness of the drug
   d. Skipping doses minimizes adverse reactions because the body has time to recover between doses
   e. None of the above

7. Patients taking theophylline _____.
   a. should not drink coffee before having a theophylline blood level drawn
   b. should be monitored for toxicity
   c. may miss doses since the drug levels are stable once established
   d. can be pregnant with no risk to the fetus
   e. Both a and b

8. In which of the following patients would administration of a xanthine derivative be contraindicated?
   a. A patient with a peptic ulcer
   b. A pregnant patient
   c. An elderly patient (older than 60 years of age)
   d. A patient who has hypothyroidism
   e. A patient with congestive heart failure

9. Corticosteroids that are used to manage chronic asthma or allergic rhinitis generally act by _____.
   a. increasing the sensitivity of beta-2 receptors
   b. decreasing the inflammatory response
   c. making the beta-2 receptor agonist drugs more effective
   d. Both a and c
   e. Answers a, b, and c

10. Which of the following drugs inhibit the production of leukotrienes?
    a. montelukast
    b. zileuton
    c. cromolyn
    d. zafirlukast
    e. flunisolide

11. The common adverse reaction of headache and abdominal pain can be associated with which of the following drugs?
    a. zafirlukast
    b. montelukast
    c. zileuton
    d. both a and c
    e. Answers a, b, and c

12. Mr. P has been prescribed zafirlukast. Which medications should he avoid so that his plasma level of zafirlukast is not increased because of a drug interaction?
    a. warfarin sodium
    b. theophylline
    c. aspirin
    d. propanolol
    e. erythromycin

13. Mast cell stabilizers _____.
    a. take 2 to 4 weeks to produce a therapeutic response
    b. must be discontinued gradually
    c. can enable other antiasthma drugs to be taken in a reduced dose
    d. can be used to treat exercise-induced bronchospasm
    e. All of the above

VI. RECALL FACTS

Indicate which of the following statements are facts with an F. If the statement is not a fact, leave the line blank.

ABOUT THINGS THAT DECREASE THE EFFECTIVENESS OF XANTHINE DERIVATIVES

____ 1. Citrus fruit consumption

____ 2. Charcoal-broiled foods

____ 3. Cigarettes

____ 4. Coffee, colas, or chocolate

____ 5. Isoniazid or rifampin administration

____ 6. Pregnancy and lactation

____ 7. Barbiturate administration

ABOUT TREATMENT WITH SYMPATHOMIMETICS

____ 1. Patients should not exceed recommended doses

____ 2. Tend to cause drowsiness and sedation

____ 3. May cause nervousness, insomnia, and restlessness

____ 4. Tachycardia, palpitations, and muscle tremors are normal and will pass with time

____ 5. Difficulty with urination or breathing should be reported to the health care provider.

____ 6. Salmeterol is used for acute asthma symptoms.

____ 7. The route of administration for formoterol fumarate is oral inhalation.

____ 8. The regular use of short-acting beta-2 agonists is to be continued during formoterol fumarate treatment.

VII. FILL IN THE BLANKS

Fill in the blanks using words from the list below.

sympathomimetic	xanthine derivatives	decreased	hypertension	hypotension
increased	intrinsic	mixed	extrinsic	cromolyn

1. _____ asthma results from a response to an allergen.

2. _____ asthma has both intrinsic and extrinsic factors.

3. _____ asthma results from chronic or recurrent respiratory infections, emotional upset, or exercise.

4. The two major types of bronchodilators are
_____ and _____.

5. Older adults taking sympathomimetic bronchodilators are at a(n) _____ risk for
adverse reactions.

6. Effects of oral hypoglycemics or insulin may be
_____ when administered with
epinephrine.

7. A sympathomimetic drug used concurrently with an oxytocic drug may cause severe
_____, and when given with an
MAOI may cause severe _____.

8. _____ is a mast cell stabilizer.

VIII. LIST

List the requested number of items.

1. List four symptoms of acute bronchospasm that
   make it a medical emergency.

   a. _____

   b. _____

   c. _____

   d. _____

2. List the four conditions in which sympathomimetics are used for treatment.

   a. _____

   b. _____

   c. _____

   d. _____

3. List the five conditions in which sympathomimetics are contraindicated.

   a. _____

   b. _____

   c. _____

   d. _____

   e. _____

4. List four adverse reactions of xanthine derivatives.

   a. _____

   b. _____

   c. _____

   d. _____

5. List six signs of theophylline toxicity.

   a. _____

   b. _____

   c. _____

   d. _____

   e. _____

   f. _____

6. List three ways you could suggest to help a patient
   manage the unpleasant taste of antiasthma drugs.

   a. _____

   b. _____

   c. _____

IX. CLINICAL APPLICATIONS

1. Mr. Y has been prescribed a corticosteroid inhalant
   for his respiratory disorder. As a health care worker involved in Mr. Y's care, what might you tell Mr.
   Y about his medication?

2. Mrs. W has been diagnosed with a respiratory disorder that requires the regular use of an aerosol inhalant to administer her bronchodilator. What should
   Mrs. W know about the use of this medication?

X. CASE STUDY

Mr. A., a 49 year old financial analyst, has been put on zileuton for his asthma. You are educating Mr. A. about the medication and how it will benefit his treatment plan. The following would be included in the information you might present.

1. What is the drug classification for zileuton?
   a. Leukotriene-receptor antagonist
   b. Leukotriene formation inhibitor
   c. Mast cell stabilizer
   d. Corticosteroid

2. What is the mode of action of zileuton?
   a. It decreases the formation of leukotriene
   b. It inhibits leukotriene receptor sites in the respiratory tract
   c. It inhibits the release of substances causing bronchoconstriction and inflammation from the mast cells
   d. It decreases the inflammatory process in the airways

3. Which of the following should be told to Mr. A.?
   a. Zileuton should always be used in an acute asthma attack.
   b. Zileuton may elevate liver enzymes.
   c. ALT levels are measured at certain intervals during treatment.
   d. Zileuton should never be used in an acute asthma attack.
   e. Answers b, c, and d

16

Antihistamines and Decongestants

I. MATCH THE FOLLOWING

Match the term from Column A with the correct definition from Column B.

COLUMN A

_____ 1. Antihistamine

_____ 2. Epigastric disorder

_____ 3. Expectoration

_____ 4. Histamine

COLUMN B

A. The elimination of thick, tenacious mucus from the respiratory tract by spitting it up

B. Discomfort in the abdomen

C. A substance in various body tissues, such as the heart, lungs, gastric mucosa, and skin, is produced in response to an injury

D. A drug used to counteract the effects of histamine on body organs and structures

II. MATCH THE FOLLOWING

Match the generic antihistamine or decongestant from Column A with the trade name from Column B.

COLUMN A

_____ 1. loratadine

_____ 2. diphenhydramine

_____ 3. fexofenadine

_____ 4. cetirizine

_____ 5. desloratadine

_____ 6. promethazine

_____ 7. chlorpheniramine

_____ 8. phenylephrine

_____ 9. oxymetazoline

_____ 10. pseudoephedrine

_____ 11. hydroxyzine

_____ 12. naphazoline HCl

_____ 13. tetrahydrozoline HCl

_____ 14. levocetirizine

_____ 15. clemastine fumarate

COLUMN B

A. Zyrtec

B. Benadryl

C. Chlor-Trimeton

D. Xyzal

E. Allegra

F. Phenergan

G. Afrin

H. Claritin

I. Vistaril

J. Sudafed-PE

K. Tavist

L. Clarinex

M. Privine

N. Tyzine

O. Sudafed

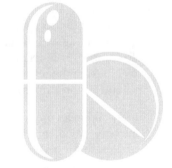

III. TRUE OR FALSE

Indicate whether each statement is True (T) or False (F).

_____ 1. Histamine release produces localized redness and swelling at the site of an injury.

_____ 2. Some antihistamines are able to prevent vomiting.

_____ 3. Antihistamines may be taken by a woman who is nursing an infant with no adverse effect to the infant.

_____ 4. Most antihistamines are administered topically.

_____ 5. Respiratory secretions may become thickened because of the use of antihistamines.

_____ 6. An adverse reaction of oral decongestants may be tachycardia and insomnia.

IV. MULTIPLE CHOICE

Circle the letter of the best answer.

1. Histamine _____.
   a. release produces an inflammatory response
   b. is released in allergic reactions
   c. is released in anaphylactic shock
   d. produces increased vasodilation and increased capillary permeability
   e. All of the above

2. Miss T is experiencing an allergic reaction to a bee sting. As a result, she might _____.
   a. need to take a histamine stimulant
   b. need to use an antihistamine
   c. go into anaphylactic shock
   d. Both b and c
   e. All of the above

3. Antihistamines have an action of _____.
   a. stimulating histamine receptors
   b. increasing the release of histamine by mast cells and basophils
   c. competing with histamine for receptor sites
   d. completely blocking all histamine receptor sites
   e. blocking the release of histamine by mast cells and Chlor-Trimeton basophils

4. After taking an antihistamine for several days for his seasonal allergy, Mr. J is starting to itch and has a rash on his chest. He may _____.
   a. be experiencing an adverse reaction
   b. be becoming used to the drug
   c. need to increase the dose he is taking
   d. be developing an allergy to the antihistamine
   e. None of the above

5. Which of the following is an oral nasal decongestant?
   a. loratadine
   b. promethazine
   c. cetirizine
   d. hydroxyzine
   e. phenylephrine HCl

6. Which of the following effects might Miss T experience as a result of the anticholinergic effects of her antihistamine medication?
   a. Dry mouth, nose, and throat
   b. Dizziness, fatigue, and hypotension
   c. Photosensitivity
   d. Skin rash and urticaria
   e. Anaphylactic shock

7. Nasal decongestants _____.
   a. are sympathomimetic drugs
   b. produce localized vasoconstriction
   c. come in topical or oral forms
   d. Both b and c
   e. Answers a, b, and c

8. Miss A, who is 82 years old, has been prescribed an antihistamine. Which of the following might Miss A be likely to experience as a result of this medication?
   a. Nervousness and irritability
   b. Dizziness, sedation, and hypotension
   c. Speech difficulties
   d. Anticholinergic effects
   e. Both b and d

9. Of the following patients, which one is not a candidate for a decongestant?
   a. A patient taking a MAOI
   b. A hypotensive patient
   c. A patient with severe coronary artery disease
   d. Both a and c
   e. Decongestant use is contraindicated in all of these patients

10. Mrs. S is experiencing rebound nasal congestion as a result of overuse. What might you suggest to her to minimize the adverse reaction?

    a. Stop using the nasal decongestants immediately
    b. Continue using the nasal decongestants as often as needed, as this reaction will go away in time
    c. Gradually discontinue use in one nostril and then the other
    d. Decrease use in both the nostrils by 1 time per day
    e. She is now addicted and will always need to use the nasal decongestant

V. FILL IN THE BLANKS

Fill in the blanks using words from the list below.

hypertension	heart disease	naphazoline
antiemetic	antipruritic	contraindicated
nasal decongestant	MAOI	stinging sensation

antihistamines	drowsiness	sedation
topical	oral	

1. Antihistamines may have additional effects such as _____, _____, or sedative effects.

2. Common adverse reactions of many antihistamines are _____ and _____.

3. Antihistamines are _____ in lactating women since the drugs pass readily into the breast milk.

4. _____ should not be taken by patients with lower respiratory tract diseases, including asthma.

5. _____ application of decongestants is more effective than the _____ route for nasal congestion relief.

6. _____ is contraindicated in patients with glaucoma.

7. Use of a(n) _____ along with a(n) _____ may cause a hypertensive crisis.

8. Nonprescription nasal decongestants should not be used by patients with _____ or _____ unless approved by their health care provider.

9. After using a topical nasal decongestant, some patients may experience a mild _____, which usually disappears with continued use.

VI. LIST

List the requested number of items.

1. List eight uses of antihistamines.

    a. _____
    b. _____
    c. _____
    d. _____
    e. _____
    f. _____
    g. _____
    h. _____

2. List five types of patients in whom antihistamines are used with caution.

    a. _____
    b. _____
    c. _____
    d. _____
    e. _____

3. List six uses of decongestants.

a. _____   d. _____

b. _____   e. _____

c. _____   f. _____

VII. CLINICAL APPLICATIONS

1. Explain to Miss E why overusing of nasal decongestant can lead to rebound nasal congestion.

2. To help Mr. W get the maximum benefit from using a decongestant, what should you, as his health care worker, be sure that he knows about this medication?

VIII. CASE STUDY

Susan Jones, age 29, has just been stung by a bee. She has a history of having stings in the past and has experienced mild-to-moderate allergic reactions. She has gone to the ambulatory clinic to seek medical care.

1. What oral medication may be prescribed for her?

   a. cetirizine
   b. chlorpheniramine maleate
   c. clemastine fumarate
   d. Any of the above

2. What are the most common side effects of these medications?

   a. Drowsiness and sedation
   b. Dizziness, disturbed coordination, and fatigue
   c. Nausea, vomiting, and diarrhea
   d. Both a and b
   e. All of the above

3. Susan's health care provider needs to assess her health history before an antihistamine is prescribed. What conditions would warrant the drug being prescribed with caution?

   a. Bronchial asthma
   b. Cardiovascular disease
   c. Hypertension
   d. Impaired kidney function
   e. All of the above

17

Antitussives, Mucolytics, and Expectorants

I. MATCH THE FOLLOWING

Match the term from Column A with the correct definition from Column B.

COLUMN A

_____ 1. Auscultating
_____ 2. Mucolytic
_____ 3. Nebulization
_____ 4. Antitussive
_____ 5. Productive cough

COLUMN B

A. A drug used to relieve coughing
B. Dispersing of a liquid medication in a mist
C. Listening for sounds within the body
D. Cough that expels secretions from the lower respiratory tract
E. A drug that loosens respiratory secretions

II. MATCH THE FOLLOWING

Match the generic drug from Column A with the trade name from Column B.

COLUMN A

_____ 1. diphenhydramine HCl
_____ 2. acetylcysteine
_____ 3. potassium iodide
_____ 4. dextromethorphan HBr and benzocaine
_____ 5. benzonatate
_____ 6. guaifenesin

COLUMN B

A. Sucrets
B. SSKI
C. Mucinex
D. Tessalon Perles
E. Benadryl
F. Mucomyst

III. MATCH THE FOLLOWING

Match the trade name of the drug from Column A with the type of drug from Column B. You may use an answer more than once.

COLUMN A

____ 1. Delsym

____ 2. Tessalon Perles

____ 3. Mucomyst

____ 4. Sucrets

____ 5. Organidin NR

____ 6. Mucinex

____ 7. Benadryl

____ 8. SSKI

____ 9. Codeine sulfate

COLUMN B

A. Mucolytic

B. Expectorant

C. Narcotic antitussive

D. Nonnarcotic antitussive

IV. TRUE OR FALSE

Indicate whether each statement is True (T) or False (F).

____ 1. To treat the discomfort of upper respiratory tract infections only an antitussive should be used.

____ 2. A peripherally acting antitussive acts by depressing the cough center located in the medulla.

____ 3. Antitussives are used to relieve only a nonproductive cough.

____ 4. A patient with a productive cough should be examined by a health care provider before starting any antitussive therapy.

____ 5. An antitussive that contains an antihistamine may have drowsiness as an adverse reaction.

____ 6. A mucolytic increases the production of respiratory secretions.

____ 7. Mucolytics are mainly administered through nebulization.

V. MULTIPLE CHOICE

Circle the letter of the best answer.

1. An example of a centrally acting antitussive is _____.

   a. benzonatate
   b. potassium iodide
   c. dextromethorphan
   d. guaifenesin
   e. terpin hydrate

2. A peripherally acting antitussive _____.

   a. acts by anesthetizing stretch receptors in the respiratory passageways
   b. acts by depressing the cough center in the medulla
   c. acts by loosening respiratory secretions
   d. helps to raise thick, tenacious mucus from the respiratory tract
   e. None of the above

3. Miss T has had a productive cough for 12 days. She has been taking Vicks Formula 44 Cough for 8 days with no relief. What action might you suggest for her?

   a. Increase the dose of her current antitussive
   b. Buy an antitussive that also contains a mucolytic
   c. Change brands of antitussives
   d. Consult with her health care provider
   e. Stop taking all medicines; she is having a rebound reaction to the antitussive

4. A patient with a productive cough who is taking an antitussive may experience _____.
   a. a pooling of secretions in the lungs
   b. pneumonia and atelectasis
   c. an increased cough reflex
   d. Both a and b
   e. All of the above

5. Expectorants _____.
   a. increase the production of respiratory secretions
   b. decrease the viscosity of mucus
   c. help raise secretions from respiratory passages
   d. should be taken with plenty of water
   e. All of the above

6. When potassium iodide is given as an expectorant to a patient who is also taking a potassium sparing diuretic, what may occur as a result of a drug interaction?
   a. Hyperkalemia, cardiac arrhythmia, or arrest
   b. Hypothyroidism
   c. Masking of a medical condition
   d. Neither drug will work; they counteract each other
   e. Both the drugs will work better

7. Before a patient is given a mucolytic or an expectorant, he or she must be assessed for _____.
   a. lung sounds
   b. dyspnea
   c. consistency of sputum
   d. description of sputum
   e. All of the above

VI. FILL IN THE BLANKS

Fill in the blanks using words from the list below.

mucolytic   potassium iodide   additive   dextromethorphan   antitussive   codeine
acetylcysteine   expectorants

1. Using a(n) _____ for a productive cough is often contraindicated.

2. When _____ is administered with MAOIs, patients may experience hypotension, fever, nausea, jerking motions of the leg, or coma.

3. Antitussives containing _____ are classified as controlled substance, schedule V.

4. Central nervous system depressants and alcohol may cause _____ depressant effects when administered with antitussives containing codeine.

5. _____ has an additional use in preventing liver damage caused by acetaminophen overdosage.

6. The expectorant _____ is contraindicated during pregnancy.

7. No significant interactions have been reported when _____ are used as directed with the exception of iodine products.

8. _____ drugs can be used as effective adjunctive therapy in cystic fibrosis and in tracheostomy care.

VII. LIST

List the requested number of items.

1. List four conditions in which antitussive containing codeine is used with caution.

   a. _____

   b. _____

   c. _____

   d. _____

2. List four examples of uses of mucolytics.

   a. _____

   b. _____

   c. _____

   d. _____

VIII. CLINICAL APPLICATIONS

1. Mr. Z is taking an antitussive with codeine at home as part of the treatment of his respiratory disorder. What should Mr. Z and his family be aware of regarding this type of medication?

2. Miss P has been prescribed the expectorant Mucinex for her respiratory problem. What are the possible adverse reactions with this medication that she should be aware of?

IX. CASE STUDY

Mr. Smith, age 59, was diagnosed with emphysema 10 years ago. He has been careful with following his care regimen and avoiding public areas during the cold and flu season. Mr. Smith recently visited his daughter and grandchildren, who were recovering from a respiratory illness. Within a week after returning home Mr. Smith developed a dry, persistent, nonproductive cough. His physician ordered benzonatate for his cough.

1. What possible symptoms of adverse reaction that he may experience?

    a. Hypotension
    b. Sedation
    c. Headache
    d. Mild dizziness
    e. Answers b, c, and d

2. Mr. Smith's cough quickly progressed to a productive cough. Because of his emphysema, the physician changed his medication to _____.

    a. a mucolytic
    b. an expectorant
    c. a narcotic antitussive
    d. a nonnarcotic antitussive
    e. Both a and b
    f. Both b and d

3. Mr. Smith is taking acetylcysteine. What are the important care aspects, about acetylcysteine, should the health care provider be aware of?

    a. It is given primarily by nebulization
    b. It is used cautiously in those with severe respiratory insufficiency or asthma
    c. It is used cautiously in older adults and debilitated adults
    d. All of the above

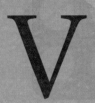

18

Cardiotonic and Miscellaneous Inotropic Drugs

I. MATCH THE FOLLOWING

Match the term from Column A with the correct definition from Column B.

COLUMN A

_____ 1. Atrial fibrillation

_____ 2. Digitalization

_____ 3. Ejection fraction

_____ 4. Positive inotropic action

COLUMN B

A. The amount of blood that the ventricle ejects per beat in relationship to the amount of blood available to eject

B. A cardiac arrhythmia characterized by rapid contractions of the atrial myocardium, resulting in an irregular and often rapid ventricular rate

C. The increased force of the contraction of the heart muscle through the use of cardiotonic drugs

D. A series of doses given until the digitalis drug begins to exert a full therapeutic effect

---

II. MATCH THE FOLLOWING

Indicate whether the drug from Column A would cause an increase or a decrease in the digitalis plasma level (Column B) of a patient. You may use an answer more than once.

COLUMN A

_____ 1. aminoglycosides

_____ 2. Macrolides

_____ 3. Benzodiazepines

_____ 4. antacids

_____ 5. Quinidine

_____ 6. st. John's wort

_____ 7. activated charcoal

_____ 8. Tetracycline

COLUMN B

A. Increase in digitalis plasma level

B. Decrease in digitalis plasma level

III. TRUE OR FALSE

Indicate whether each statement is True (T) or False (F).

____ 1. Cardiotonics are used to improve the efficiency and contraction of the heart muscle.

____ 2. Digitalis glycosides is an another term for a cardiotonic drugs.

____ 3. Positive inotropic action results in increased cardiac output and decreased heart rate.

____ 4. Normal doses of a cardiotonic drug may cause toxic drug effects.

____ 5. Hypokalemia is a concern for patients receiving digoxin immune Fab.

____ 6. A patient receiving a miscellaneous inotropic drug must have continuous cardiac monitoring.

____ 7. Renal function in patients taking cardiotonics is not a consideration since the drug is metabolized by the liver.

IV. MULTIPLE CHOICE

Circle the letter of the best answer.

1. The most commonly used cardiotonic drug is
   ____.
   a. lidocaine HCl
   b. digoxin
   c. tocainide HCl
   d. esmolol HCl
   e. acebutolol

2. Cardiotonics are used to treat ____.
   a. heart failure
   b. ventricular fibrillation
   c. atrial fibrillation
   d. Both a and b
   e. Both a and c

3. Mrs. Q is receiving digitalis for her heart failure. If she mentions ____, the health care worker should notify the health care provider immediately.
   a. blurred vision
   b. anorexia
   c. headache
   d. abnormal heart beat
   e. All of the above

4. Which of the following drugs is more often used in the short-term management of severe heart failure that is not controlled by digitalis?
   a. Digoxin immune Fab
   b. Milrinone
   c. Esmolol
   d. Thiazide
   e. Inamrinone

5. Miscellaneous inotropic drugs such as inamrinone or milrinone ____.
   a. cure heart failure
   b. help manage arrhythmias
   c. control the signs and symptoms of heart failure
   d. decrease cardiac output
   e. prevent right-sided ventricular failure

6. Mr. T was accidentally given a double dose of digoxin at the hospital. To treat this potentially life-threatening toxicity, the health care provider may need to ____.
   a. withdraw the drug from his next scheduled treatment regimen
   b. change his medicine
   c. order digoxin immune Fab
   d. Both a and c
   e. Both a and b

7. Digitalization of a patient ____.
   a. involves a series of doses
   b. includes a first dose of approximately half of the total dose
   c. may involve injections or tablets
   d. Both a and b
   e. Answers a, b, and c

8. It is important that family members and patients undergoing long-term cardiotonic therapy ____.
   a. understand the need to take the drug as prescribed
   b. take their pulse as directed
   c. are aware of drug interactions
   d. follow dietary recommendations
   e. All of the above

9. All of the following are symptoms of left ventricular dysfunction except
    a. shortness of breath with exercise.
    b. dry, hacking cough or wheezing.
    c. orthopnea.
    d. restlessness and anxiety.
    e. All of the above

10. Central nervous system signs and symptoms of digitalis toxicity include
    a. headache.
    b. apathy.
    c. numbness of the extremities.
    d. Both a and b

11. Adverse reactions seen with inamrinone lactate include
    a. arrhythmias.
    b. hypotension.
    c. nausea.
    d. hepatotoxicity.
    e. All of the above

12. Which of the following is not true about digoxin immune Fab?
    a. It is an antidote for digoxin toxicity
    b. The dosage depends on the serum digoxin level or estimate of the amount of digoxin ingested to be neutralized
    c. The drug improves heart failure symptoms
    d. The drug is administered over 30 minutes.

V. RECALL FACTS

Indicate which of the following statements are facts with an F. If the statement is not a fact, leave the line blank.

ABOUT PATIENT ASSESSMENT BEFORE CARDIOTONIC THERAPY

_____ 1. Blood pressure, pulse, and respiratory rate

_____ 2. Lung sounds and appearance of sputum

_____ 3. Height and sex of patient

_____ 4. Weight

_____ 5. Presence of edema

_____ 6. Jugular vein distention

_____ 7. Environment patient works in

_____ 8. Availability of medical care

VI. FILL IN THE BLANKS

Fill in the blanks using words from the list below. Words may be used more than once.

hypokalemia	rapid	hypomagnesemia	slowed	same	decreased
rapid	beta blockers	short	ACE inhibitors	diuretics	gradual

1. The first three lines of treatment for heart failure are _____, _____, and _____.

2. Digoxin has a(n) _____ onset and a(n) _____ duration of action.

3. When a cardiotonic is taken with food, absorption is _____ but the amount of drug absorbed is the _____, unless it is taken with a high-fiber meal; then absorption may be _____.

4. Two methods of digitalization may be used when a patient starts treatment with a cardiotonic—the _____ method or the _____ method.

5. Patients receiving a cardiotonic drug and a diuretic are at risk for _____ and _____.

VII. LIST

List the requested number of items.

1. List two ways in which cardiotonics act.

   a. _____

   b. _____

2. List four factors that influence the dose of cardio-tonics that a patient may receive.

   a. _____

   b. _____

   c. _____

   d. _____

3. List four systems that may show signs of digitalis toxicity.

   a. _____

   b. _____

   c. _____

   d. _____

4. List four conditions in which a cardiotonic is contraindicated.

   a. _____

   b. _____

   c. _____

   d. _____

VIII. CLINICAL APPLICATIONS

1. Mrs. K will be continuing her cardiotonic drug therapy at home after her discharge. As the health care worker assigned to her discharge, what important points should you make sure that she understands about this type of medication?

2. You suspect that Mr. Q has right-sided ventricular heart failure. What symptoms would you expect to observe in Mr. Q as his disease progresses?

IX. CASE STUDY

Mrs. Black's health care provider has decided that she has heart failure and that she would benefit from a cardiotonic medication. Before the therapy is started she will be assessed to establish a database for comparison during therapy.

1. The physical assessment should include
   a. blood pressure, apical-radial pulse, and respiratory rate.
   b. lung sounds.
   c. examining the extremities for edema.
   d. checking the jugular veins for distention.
   e. measuring weight.
   f. Answers a, b, and d
   g. All of the above.

2. Mrs. Black is going to be digitalized. This may be accomplished by
   a. rapid digitalization (administering a loading dose).
   b. slow digitalization (administering an increased dose each week for a month).
   c. gradual digitalization (giving a maintenance dose allowing the body to gradually accumulate therapeutic blood levels).
   d. Both a and c

3. The dose of digoxin which Mrs. Black receives will be determined by
   a. her renal function.
   b. age.
   c. other medications.
   d. All of the above

19

Antiarrhythmic Drugs

I. MATCH THE FOLLOWING

Match the term from Column A with the correct definition from Column B.

COLUMN A

____ 1. Arrhythmia

____ 2. Cinchonism

____ 3. Proarrhythmic effect

____ 4. Refractory period

COLUMN B

A. The development of a new arrhythmia or the worsening of an existing arrhythmia caused by an antiarrhythmic drug

B. A term for quinidine toxicity

C. The period between transmissions of nerve impulses along a nerve fiber

D. A disturbance or irregularity in the heart rate or the rhythm, or both

II. MATCH THE FOLLOWING

Match the generic drug form Column A with the trade name from Column B.

COLUMN A

____ 1. flecainide

____ 2. digoxin

____ 3. disopyramide

____ 4. esmolol

____ 5. propafenone

____ 6. amiodarone

____ 7. dronedarone

____ 8. acebutolol

____ 9. dofetilide

COLUMN B

A. Cordarone

B. Norpace

C. Lanoxin

D. Sectral

E. Multaq

F. Rythmol

G. Tikosyn

H. Brevibloc

I. Tambocor

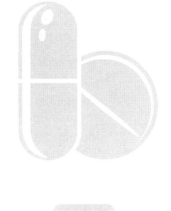

III. MATCH THE FOLLOWING

Match the class I drug from Column A with the correct subclass from Column B. You may use an answer more than once.

COLUMN A

____ 1. propafenone
____ 2. quinidine
____ 3. procainamide
____ 4. flecainide
____ 5. disopyramide
____ 6. lidocaine

COLUMN B

A. Class IA
B. Class IB
C. Class IC

IV. MATCH THE FOLLOWING

Match the drug from Column A with the class from Column B. You may use an answer more than once.

COLUMN A

____ 1. lidocaine
____ 2. acebutolol
____ 3. quinidine sulfate
____ 4. esmolol
____ 5. propafenone
____ 6. flecainide
____ 7. ibutilide
____ 8. amiodarone
____ 9. verapamil
____ 10. diltiazem
____ 11. dofetilide

COLUMN B

A. Class I
B. Class II
C. Class III
D. Class IV

V. TRUE OR FALSE

Indicate whether each statement is True (T) or False (F).

____ 1. The goal of antiarrhythmic drug therapy is to inhibit normal cardiac function and to prevent a life-threatening cardiac rhythm.

____ 2. Lidocaine works by reducing the number of stimuli that can pass along myocardial fibers, which decreases the pulse rate and corrects the arrhythmia.

____ 3. Ibutilide and dofetilide are used to convert atrial fibrillation or atrial flutter back to sinus rhythm.

____ 4. Class IV antiarrhythmic drugs are also called calcium channel blockers.

____ 5. Propranolol may sometimes be used to treat migraine headaches.

____ 6. Antiarrhythmic drugs never cause new arrhythmias.

____ 7. Proarrhythmic effects of a drug are easy to distinguish from a pre-existing arrhythmia.

VI. MULTIPLE CHOICE

Circle the letter of the best answer.

1. Antiarrhythmic drugs are classified _____.
   a. according to their effects on the action potential of cardiac cells
   b. according to their presumed mechanism of action
   c. based on their chemical components
   d. based on their effects on the muscular tissue of the heart
   e. Both a and b

2. Which class of antiarrhythmic drug has a membrane-stabilizing effect on the cells of the myocardium?
   a. Class I
   b. Class II
   c. Class III
   d. Class IV
   e. None of the above

3. An example of an antiarrhythmic that acts by decreasing the rate of diastolic depolarization in the ventricles and increases the fiber threshold is _____.
   a. disopyramide
   b. quinidine
   c. procainamide
   d. lidocaine
   e. verapamil

4. Which of the following drugs works by raising the threshold of the ventricular myocardium?
   a. quinidine
   b. procainamide
   c. verapamil
   d. lidocaine
   e. esmolol

5. Which class of antiarrhythmic acts by having a direct stabilizing action on the myocardium?
   a. Class IA
   b. Class IB
   c. Class IC
   d. Class II
   e. Class III

6. Class II antiarrhythmic drugs work by _____.
   a. shortening the refractory period
   b. blocking stimulation of beta receptors of the heart

   c. stimulating alpha receptors
   d. shortening repolarization
   e. decreasing the threshold

7. Which of the Class III antiarrhythmic drugs selectively blocks potassium channels?
   a. ibutilide
   b. dofetilide
   c. bretylium
   d. amiodarone
   e. None of the above

8. Older adults taking antiarrhythmics are at increased risk for _____.
   a. proarrhythmias
   b. worsening of existing arrhythmias
   c. hypotension
   d. congestive heart failure
   e. All of the above

9. Cinchonism may be indicated by all of the following symptoms except _____.
   a. tinnitus and vertigo
   b. hearing loss
   c. headache and light-headedness
   d. nausea
   e. All of the above

10. An adverse reaction of disopyramide is urinary retention. This is caused by _____.
   a. beta-adrenergic stimulation
   b. anticholinergic effects
   c. cholinergic blocking effects
   d. beta-adrenergic blocking effects
   e. None of the above

11. Dofetilide is not given with cimetidine because _____.
   a. dofetilide levels may increase by 50%
   b. cimetidine levels may increase by 50%
   c. dofetilide levels may decrease by 50%
   d. cimetidine levels may decrease by 50%
   e. Both a and b

VII. RECALL FACTS

Indicate which of the following statements are facts with an F. If the statement is not a fact, leave the line blank.

ABOUT PATIENT ASSESSMENT BEFORE ANTIARRHYTHMIC THERAPY

____ 1. Blood pressure, pulse, and respiratory rate

____ 2. Weight

____ 3. Urinary output

____ 4. Cardiac monitoring available

____ 5. ECG

____ 6. Lab tests

VIII. FILL IN THE BLANKS

Fill in the blanks using words from the list below.

additive
acebutolol
cinchonism

quinidine
esmolol
Xylocaine

procainamide
propranolol
verapamil

proarrhythmia effect
repolarization
class I-C drugs

1. When two antiarrhythmic drugs are given concurrently, the patient may experience _____ effects.

2. When _____ and _____ are administered with digitalis, the risk of digitalis toxicity is increased.

3. When an antiarrhythmic drug causes a new arrhythmia or worsens existing arrhythmias, this is called _____.

4. Quinidine toxicity is called _____.

5. _____, _____, and _____ are examples of Class II antiarrhythmic drugs.

6. _____ is the movement back to the original state of positive and negative ions after a stimulus passes along a nerve fiber.

7. Another name for lidocaine is _____.

8. _____ have a direct stabilizing action on the myocardium.

9. _____ is used cautiously in patients with a history of serious ventricular arrhythmias or CHF.

IX. LIST

List the requested number of items.

1. List four arrhythmic conditions in which antiarrhythmic drugs could be used.

   a. _____

   b. _____

   c. _____

   d. _____

2. List three times when a proarrhythmic effect is more likely to occur.

   a. _____

   b. _____

   c. _____

3. List five antiarrhythmic drugs that may cause agranulocytosis.

a. _____

b. _____

c. _____

d. _____

e. _____

4. List four conditions in which antiarrhythmic drugs are contraindicated.

a. _____

b. _____

c. _____

d. _____

X. CLINICAL APPLICATIONS

1. Mr. M. is starting on an antiarrhythmic medication. What are the key points he and his family should be aware of?

2. You suspect that Mr. G. may have cinchonism. What are the signs and symptoms that may be present?

XI. CASE STUDY

Mr. Jones, age 57, has recently started taking dronedarone for his atrial fibrillation. He and his family are being taught about this new medication.

1. What dietary precautions should he be told about?
   a. Avoid spinach
   b. Do not take the medication with grapefruit juice
   c. Always take the medication with milk
   d. None of the above

2. You are reviewing Mr. Jones' current medication list to see if there are potential drug interaction problems. Dronedarone may have an additive effect with
   a. beta blockers.
   b. calcium channel blockers.
   c. class I antiarrhythmics.
   d. class III antiarrhythmics.
   e. All of the above

3. Mr. Jones needs to let you know if he is having adverse reactions from taking dronedarone. Which of the following are adverse reactions for him to be aware of?
   a. Abdominal pain
   b. Asthenia
   c. Diarrhea
   d. Nausea and vomiting
   e. All of the above

20

Antianginal and Peripheral Vasodilating Drugs

I. MATCH THE FOLLOWING

Match the term from Column A with the correct definition from Column B.

COLUMN A

_____ 1. Angina

_____ 2. Intermittent claudication

_____ 3. Lumen

_____ 4. Prophylaxis

_____ 5. Transdermal system

COLUMN B

A. A group of symptoms characterized by pain in the calf muscle of one or both legs.

B. Prevention

C. A convenient form of drug administration in which the drug is impregnated in a pad and absorbed through the skin

D. A disorder that causes decreased oxygen supply to the heart muscle and results in chest pain or pressure

E. The inside diameter of a vessel

II. MATCH THE FOLLOWING

Match the generic nitroglycerin drugs from Column A with the trade name from Column B.

COLUMN A

_____ 1. nitroglycerin translingual

_____ 2. nitroglycerin sublingual

_____ 3. nitroglycerin sustained release

_____ 4. nitroglycerin topical

_____ 5. nitroglycerin transdermal system

COLUMN B

A. Nitrostat

B. Minitran

C. Nitro-Bid

D. Nitro-Time

E. Nitrolingual

III. MATCH THE FOLLOWING

Match the generic calcium channel blocker from in Column A with the trade name from Column B.

COLUMN A

_____ 1. diltiazem

_____ 2. nicardipine

_____ 3. nifedipine

_____ 4. verapamil

_____ 5. amlodipine

COLUMN B

A. Cardizem

B. Calan

C. Cardene

D. Procardia

E. Norvasc

IV. MATCH THE FOLLOWING

Match the antianginal or peripheral vasodilating generic drug from Column A with the trade name from Column B.

COLUMN A

____ 1. cilostazol

____ 2. isosorbide mononitrate, oral

____ 3. isosorbide dinitrate, oral

____ 4. isosorbide dinitrate, sublingual

COLUMN B

A. Isordil

B. Dilatrate-SR

C. ISMO

D. Pletal

V. TRUE OR FALSE

Indicate whether each statement is True (T) or False (F).

____ 1. Antianginal drugs work by causing peripheral vasodilation.

____ 2. Nitrate drugs work by having a direct relaxing effect on the smooth muscle layer of blood vessels.

____ 3. Nitrates are used to treat angina pectoris.

____ 4. Oral nitroglycerin may be swallowed without regard to meals.

____ 5. Patients using nitroglycerin for long-term treatment can develop a tolerance to the drug.

____ 6. The effect of calcium channel blockers is the same as the effect of nitrates.

____ 7. Adverse reactions to calcium channel blockers are frequently severe and often require discontinuation of the drug.

____ 8. Rebound angina is probably caused by an increase in calcium ions flowing into cells causing coronary artery spasm.

____ 9. Patients taking calcium channel blockers should be watched for signs of congestive heart failure.

____ 10. Peripheral vasodilating drugs show conclusively that they increase blood flow to ischemic areas of the body.

____ 11. Patients taking peripheral vasodilating drugs may see no significant improvement for several weeks after the therapy had begun.

VI. MULTIPLE CHOICE

Circle the letter of the best answer.

1. Which of the following drugs is used to treat Raynaud's disease?

   a. cilostazol
   b. isoxsuprine
   c. nifedipine
   d. papaverine
   e. diltiazem

2. Peripheral vasodilating drugs act to ____.

   a. inhibit platelet aggregation
   b. relieve the pain of angina
   c. increase calcium ion concentration in the cells
   d. reduce inflammation
   e. block alpha-adrenergic nerves and stimulate beta-adrenergic nerves

3. Pletal has a generic name of ____.

   a. cilostazol
   b. isoxsuprine HCl
   c. papaverine HCl
   d. verapamil HCl
   e. amyl nitrate

4. Because of the action of peripheral vasodilating drugs, which adverse reaction might you anticipate in a patient?

   a. Dysuria
   b. Hypertension
   c. Hypotension
   d. Dry mouth
   e. Paleness

5. Mrs. C has been taking a peripheral vasodilating drug regularly for several weeks for a peripheral vascular disorder. What signs might Mrs. C begin to note that would indicate an improvement in her condition?

   a. A decrease in pain
   b. An increase in warmth of extremities
   c. A stronger peripheral pulse
   d. Changes in the color of her extremities
   e. All of the Above

6. L-arginine should be used with caution by patients who have _____.

   a. congestive heart failure
   b. hypertension
   c. angina
   d. sickle cell anemia
   e. been taking MAOIs

7. Mr. V has called the office and said that his episode of chest pain has not responded to three doses of nitroglycerin given every 5 minutes for 15 minutes. What might you tell him to do?

   a. Take another dose and call back in 15 minutes
   b. Increase the dose and try it three more times in 15 minutes
   c. Try chewing the tablets instead of placing them under the tongue
   d. Notify his health care provider immediately
   e. None of the above

8. Antianginal drugs include the _____.

   a. phosphodiesterase II inhibitors
   b. nitrates
   c. adrenergic blocking agents
   d. calcium channel blockers
   e. Both b and d

9. Nitrates _____.

   a. increase the lumen of the artery
   b. increase the volume of blood flow
   c. increase the oxygen supply to the cardiac tissue
   d. decrease chest pain or pressure
   e. All of the above

10. A common adverse reaction of nitrate administration is _____.

    a. vomiting
    b. headache
    c. diarrhea
    d. dry mouth
    e. CNS stimulation

11. In which of the following conditions are the nitrates contraindicated?

    a. Renal failure
    b. Closed-angle glaucoma
    c. Cirrhosis
    d. Leukemia
    e. Orthostatic hypotension

12. The transdermal system of nitroglycerin administration has better results when the patient _____.

    a. applies the patch at the same location repeatedly
    b. leaves the patch on for 10 to 14 hours
    c. rubs the patch on the skin
    d. places the patch on a mucous membrane
    e. wets the patch before application

13. Calcium channel blockers are used to _____.

    a. prevent anginal pain
    b. treat vasospastic angina
    c. treat chronic stable angina
    d. stop anginal pain once started
    e. Answers a, b, and c

14. Mr. F is an 85-year-old man taking an antianginal drug. What should his health care provider watch for to minimize his risk of injury?

    a. Dry mouth
    b. Increased postural hypotension
    c. Peripheral edema
    d. Skin rash
    e. Dermatitis

15. Discontinuation of a calcium channel blocker _____.

    a. may cause an increase in chest pain
    b. should be done gradually
    c. may cause rebound angina
    d. may cause coronary arteries to spasm
    e. All of the above

VII. RECALL FACTS

Indicate which of the following statements are facts with an F. If the statement is not a fact, leave the line blank.

ABOUT CONTRAINDICATIONS, PRECAUTIONS, AND INTERACTIONS OF CALCIUM CHANNEL BLOCKERS

____ 1. They are contraindicated in pregnancy and during lactation

____ 2. They are contraindicated in patients who have sick sinus syndrome

____ 3. They are contraindicated in patients with second- or third-degree AV block

____ 4. Effects are decreased when given with cimetidine or ranitidine

____ 5. They have an antiplatelet effect when given with aspirin

____ 6. They may increase a patient's risk for digitalis toxicity when give with digoxin

ABOUT PATIENT MANAGEMENT ISSUES WITH NITRATES

____ 1. With treatment, angina should decrease in frequency or be eliminated

____ 2. A dry mouth will decrease the absorption of sublingual or buccal forms of the drug

____ 3. They may be administered in a topical form

____ 4. Patients never develop a tolerance to nitroglycerin

____ 5. Oral nitroglycerin should be taken on an empty stomach

VIII. FILL IN THE BLANKS

Fill in the blanks using words from the list below. You may use an answer more than once.

hypotensive	disappear	increased	decreased	Isordil
Nitrostat	intermittent claudication	pulse rate	gradual	

1. _____ is used for prevention and long-term treatment of angina, whereas _____ is used to relieve the pain of acute anginal attacks.

2. A(n) _____ hypotensive effect may be seen when nitrates are administered with antihypertensives or alcohol, whereas a(n) _____ effect of heparin may be exhibited if IV nitroglycerin is administered.

3. The effects of calcium channel blockers are _____ when given with cimetidine or ranitidine, but are _____ when given with phenobarbital or phenytoin.

4. Older adults may have a greater _____ effect while taking antianginal drugs than younger adults.

5. Most adverse reactions of antianginal drugs will _____ after a period of time.

6. A manifestation of peripheral vascular disease in which other atherosclerotic lesions develop in the leg and cause pain in the calf muscle may lead to _____.

7. Peripheral vasodilating drugs can cause a physiological increase in the _____.

8. Improvement will be _____ in the treatment of peripheral vascular disease.

IX. LIST

List the requested number of items.

1. List the four forms of nitrate administration.

   a. _____

   b. _____

   c. _____

   d. _____

2. List four common adverse reactions to calcium channel blockers.

   a. _____

   b. _____

   c. _____

   d. _____

3. List three disorders in which a peripheral vasodilating drug may be used.

   a. _____

   b. _____

   c. _____

4. List four conditions that the herbal supplement L-arginine is marketed to improve or prevent.

   a. _____

   b. _____

   c. _____

   d. _____

X. CLINICAL APPLICATIONS

1. Mr. B is taking a peripheral vasodilating drug. Give Mr. B a short explanation about how these drugs may work to relieve some or all of his symptoms.

2. Explain Miss T how to administer her sublingual or buccal nitrate medication.

XI. CASE STUDY

Mr. Jones, age 72, has been diagnosed with angina. His doctor has prescribed verapamil and PRN nitroglycerin sublingual.

1. What are the possible adverse events that may occur with the use of verapamil?

   a. Dizziness
   b. Constipation
   c. Hypotension
   d. Headache
   e. All of the above

2. Mr. Jones is at home, just had a large meal. He is experiencing chest pain. He has taken nitroglycerin 3 times, 15 minutes apart. What should he do now?

   a. Take one more SL nitro
   b. Take an extra verapamil
   c. Call his health care provider
   d. Take a nap

3. Mr. Jones' medications have been changed to include nitroglycerin ointment. Which of the following would you include when you instruct him about the use of this medication?

   a. Do not rub the medication into the skin
   b. Do not allow the medication to come into contact with fingers or hands
   c. Apply the medication to the same site daily
   d. Both a and b

21

Antihypertensive Drugs

I. MATCH THE FOLLOWING

Match the term from Column A with the correct definition from Column B.

COLUMN A

____ 1. Aldosterone

____ 2. Endogenous

____ 3. Hypertension

____ 4. Isolated systolic hypertension

____ 5. Malignant hypertension

____ 6. Secondary hypertension

COLUMN B

A. A condition of only an elevated systolic pressure

B. A systolic pressure greater than 140 mm Hg and a diastolic pressure greater than 90 mm Hg

C. Hypertension in which a direct cause can be identified

D. A hormone that promotes the retention of sodium and water, which may contribute to a rise in blood pressure

E. Hypertension in which the diastolic pressure usually exceeds 130 mm Hg

F. Substances normally manufactured by the body

II. MATCH THE FOLLOWING

Match the ACE inhibitor or angiotensin receptor antagonist generic drug from Column A with the trade name in Column B.

COLUMN A

____ 1. irbesartan

____ 2. ramipril

____ 3. lisinopril

____ 4. losartan

____ 5. valsartan

____ 6. candesartan

____ 7. benazepril

____ 8. quinapril

____ 9. moexipril

____ 10. enalapril

____ 11. perindopril

____ 12. trandolapril

____ 13. azilsartan

____ 14. eprosartan

____ 15. telmisartan

COLUMN B

A. Prinivil

B. Diovan

C. Atacand

D. Avapro

E. Cozaar

F. Lotensin

G. Altace

H. Vasotec

I. Accupril

J. Univasc

K. Mavik

L. Micardis

M. Teveten

N. Edarbi

O. Aceon

III. MATCH THE FOLLOWING

Match the drug from Column A with the type of drug from Column B. You may use an answer more than once.

COLUMN A	COLUMN B
____ 1. enalapril	A. ACE inhibitor
____ 2. perindopril	B. Angiotensin II receptor antagonist
____ 3. eprosartan	
____ 4. irbesartan	
____ 5. telmisartan	
____ 6. benazepril	
____ 7. lisinopril	
____ 8. candesartan	

IV. MATCH THE FOLLOWING

Match the generic antihypertensive drug from Column A with the trade name from Column B.

COLUMN A	COLUMN B
____ 1. penbutolol	A. Tenex
____ 2. nadolol	B. Lotensin
____ 3. acebutolol	C. Catapres
____ 4. guanfacine	D. Levatol
____ 5. epoprostenol	E. Sectral
____ 6. clonidine	F. Corgard
____ 7. doxazosin	G. Cardura
____ 8. prazosin	H. DynaCirc
____ 9. atenolol	I. Cardura
____ 10. benazepril	J. Tenormin
____ 11. isradipine	K. Minipress
____ 12. doxazosin	L. Flolan

V. MATCH THE FOLLOWING

Match the generic antihypertensive drug from Column A with the type of antihypertensive from Column B. You may use an answer more than once.

COLUMN A	COLUMN B
____ 1. reserpine	A. Peripheral vasodilator
____ 2. propranolol	B. Beta-adrenergic blocking drug
____ 3. prazosin	C. Antiadrenergic—centrally acting
____ 4. nadolol	D. Antiadrenergic—peripherally acting
____ 5. guanabenz	
____ 6. guanadrel	
____ 7. hydralazine	
____ 8. terazosin	
____ 9. acebutolol	
____ 10. methyldopa	
____ 11. bisoprolol	
____ 12. guanfacine	

VI. TRUE OR FALSE

Indicate whether each statement is True (T) or False (F).

____ 1. With proper treatment essential hypertension can be cured.

____ 2. Diuretics and beta-blocking drugs may sometimes be prescribed first for the treatment of hypertension.

____ 3. Treatment of hypertension often involves changing medications or adding a second drug to the therapy regimen.

____ 4. All antihypertensive drugs work equally well, so treatment plans are easy to establish.

____ 5. When monitoring the blood pressure of a patient receiving antihypertensive therapy, it does not matter whether the person is always in the same position.

____ 6. Hypertension occurs only in older adults.

____ 7. Older adults should be given a lower dose of nitroprusside because they seem to be more sensitive to its hypotensive effects.

VII. MULTIPLE CHOICE

Circle the letter of the best answer.

1. Which types of drugs listed below can be used to treat hypertension?
   a. Calcium channel blockers
   b. Antiadrenergic drugs
   c. ACE inhibitors
   d. Diuretics
   e. All of the above

2. ACE inhibitors lower blood pressure by _____.
   a. preventing the conversion of angiotensin I to angiotensin II
   b. preventing sodium and water retention
   c. blocking receptor sites for angiotensin II
   d. Both a and b
   e. Answers a, b, and c

3. Antihypertensive drugs _____.
   a. are used to treat hypertension
   b. may cause postural or orthostatic hypotension
   c. must be discontinued gradually over 2 to 4 days
   d. may cause the patient to become dehydrated and alter the electrolyte balance
   e. All of the above

4. Mr. G is being treated with a diuretic for his hypertension. What signs or symptoms should a health care worker be alert for?
   a. Hyponatremia
   b. Dehydration
   c. Hypokalemia
   d. Electrolyte imbalance
   e. All of the above

5. Which type of antihypertensive drug is a Pregnancy Category D during the second and third trimesters and therefore is contraindicated?
   a. Angiotensin II receptor antagonists
   b. ACE inhibitors
   c. Peripheral vasodilators
   d. Antiadrenergics–centrally acting
   e. Both a and b

6. From which of the herbal remedies or supplements listed below has it been demonstrated that hypertensive patients may benefit?
   a. Hawthorn extracts
   b. Vitamin E and aspirin
   c. Garlic and onion
   d. Ginkgo biloba
   e. All of the above

7. Mr. S is being treated for hypertension. His health care worker notes that after weighing him he has gained 3 pounds since the previous day. The health care worker should _____.
   a. keep Mr. S from drinking water
   b. report this information to the health care provider
   c. encourage Mr. S to stay with his diet
   d. ignore the information as he was wearing his shoes on the scale
   e. not worry unless his blood pressure is also higher

VIII. RECALL FACTS

Indicate which of the following statements are facts with an F. If the statement is not a fact, leave the line blank.

ABOUT LIFE STYLE CHANGES THAT REDUCE THE RISK OF HYPERTENSION

____ 1. Weight loss

____ 2. Quit smoking

____ 3. Increase fluid intake

____ 4. Eliminate carbohydrates from diet

____ 5. Reduce stress

____ 6. Increase salt consumption

____ 7. Regular aerobic exercise

____ 8. Move to a warm, dry climate

____ 9. Use an electric blanket

ABOUT INCREASED EFFECTS OF ANTIHYPERTENSIVES, ACE INHIBITORS, OR ANGIOTENSIN II RECEPTOR ANTAGONISTS

____ 1. When administered with another antihypertensive

____ 2. When administered with a diuretic

____ 3. When administered with an MAOI

____ 4. When administered with NSAID

____ 5. When administered with antacids

____ 6. When administered with phenobarbital

IX. FILL IN THE BLANKS

Fill in the blanks using words from the list below.

organ damage	sodium	gradually	high	doxazosin
metoprolol	atenolol	timolol maleate	nadolol	propranolol
lifetime	lumen	fenoldopam	nitroprusside	

1. Once essential hypertension develops, management of this disorder is a _____ task.

2. Patients with malignant hypertension experience _____ as a result of hypertension.

3. Vasodilation increases the _____ of the arterial blood vessel.

4. Diuretics increase the excretion of _____ from the body.

5. _____ and _____ are IV drugs that can be used to treat hypertensive emergencies.

6. When discontinuing an antihypertensive drug, the dosage is _____ reduced over 2 to 4 days.

7. It has been suggested that blood pressure can be lowered by a diet _____ in magnesium, calcium, and potassium.

8. _____, _____, and _____ can be used to treat angina pectoris.

9. _____ can be used to treat benign prostatic hypertrophy.

10. _____ and _____ are sometimes used to treat migraines.

X. LIST

List the requested number of items.

1. List four risk factors for hypertension.

   a. _____

   b. _____

   c. _____

   d. _____

2. List four things you could advise a patient to do to minimize his or her risk of injury from postural hypotension.

   a. _____

   b. _____

   c. _____

   d. _____

3. List the six types of drugs used to treat hypertension.

   a. _____

   b. _____

   c. _____

   d. _____

   e. _____

   f. _____

4. List four antihypertensive drugs with vasodilating activity.

   a. _____

   b. _____

   c. _____

   d. _____

5. List the two antihypertensive drugs used to treat glaucoma.

   a. _____

   b. _____

XI. CLINICAL APPLICATIONS

1. Mr. E is taking multiple drugs to treat his hypertension. His risk for orthostatic hypotension is increased because of this. What are several things that Mr. E could do to help reduce his risk of injury?

2. Mrs. P has been taking two different antihypertensive medications over the past several months, but her blood pressure still remains elevated. What might the health care provider try next to bring Mrs. P's blood pressure down?

XII. CASE STUDY

Mrs. L., age 73, has recently been diagnosed with hypertension. Her health care provider has recommended that she starts on a beta blocker medication and works on some lifestyle changes.

1. What are possible lifestyle changes her health care provider may recommend?

   a. Weight loss
   b. Increased aerobic exercise
   c. Low salt diet
   d. All of the above

2. Mrs. L. and her family receive information about taking antihypertensives when coming in for an office visit. Information given to them would include which of the following?

   a. Increase sodium intake
   b. Do not be concerned if dizziness occurs
   c. Avoid drinking alcohol
   d. None of the above

3. Mrs. L. has been prescribed captopril to control her hypertension. What adverse reactions might she experience?

   a. Peptic ulcer
   b. Pruritus
   c. Cough
   d. All of the above

22

Antihyperlipidemic Drugs

I. MATCH THE FOLLOWING

Match the term from Column A with the correct definition from Column B.

COLUMN A

_____ 1. Atherosclerosis
_____ 2. Catalyst
_____ 3. Cholesterol
_____ 4. HDL
_____ 5. Lipids
_____ 6. Lipoprotein
_____ 7. LDL
_____ 8. Triglycerides

COLUMN B

A. One of the lipids in the blood

B. A substance that accelerates a chemical reaction without undergoing a change

C. Fats or fat-like substances in the blood

D. Transports cholesterol to peripheral cells

E. A disorder in which lipid deposits accumulate on the lining of the blood vessels, eventually producing degenerative changes and obstruction of blood flow

F. A type of lipid in the blood

G. A lipid-containing protein

H. Carry cholesterol from peripheral cells to the liver

II. MATCH THE FOLLOWING

Match the generic drug from Column A with the trade name from Column B.

COLUMN A

_____ 1. cholestyramine
_____ 2. atorvastatin
_____ 3. lovastatin
_____ 4. clofibrate
_____ 5. simvastatin
_____ 6. niacin
_____ 7. fenofibrate
_____ 8. colestipol
_____ 9. fluvastatin
_____ 10. pravastatin

COLUMN B

A. Zocor
B. Lipitor
C. Mevacor
D. Prevalite
E. Atromid-S
F. Tricor
G. Lescol
H. Niaspan
I. Pravachol
J. Colestid

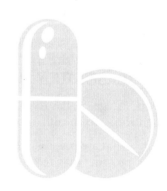

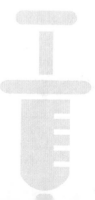

III. MATCH THE FOLLOWING

Match the drug from Column A with the type of antihyperlipidemic from Column B. You may use an answer more than once.

COLUMN A

_____ 1. colesevelam

_____ 2. atorvastatin

_____ 3. lovastatin

_____ 4. clofibrate

_____ 5. gemfibrozil

_____ 6. cholestyramine

_____ 7. simvastatin

_____ 8. fluvastatin

_____ 9. pravastatin

_____ 10. fenofibrate

_____ 11. colestipol

COLUMN B

A. Fibric acid derivatives

B. HMG-CoA reductase inhibitors

C. Bile acid sequestrants

IV. MATCH THE FOLLOWING

Match the fibric acid derivative drug from Column A with the correct action from Column B.

COLUMN A

_____ 1. clofibrate

_____ 2. fenofibrate

_____ 3. gemfibrozil

COLUMN B

A. Increases the excretion of cholesterol in the feces and decreases triglyceride production in the liver

B. Stimulates the breakdown of VLDL to LDL

C. Reduces VLDL and stimulates catabolism of triglyceride-rich lipoproteins

V. TRUE OR FALSE

Indicate whether each statement is True (T) or False (F).

_____ 1. The two lipids found in blood are cholesterol and triglycerides.

_____ 2. Lipoproteins can bind water-insoluble lipids and transport them throughout the body.

_____ 3. When the cells of the body have the cholesterol that they need, they discard the excess into the blood where it can then form atherosclerotic plaque.

_____ 4. High-density lipoprotein is considered to be the "good" lipoprotein and should be a high number.

_____ 5. In general, the higher the LDL level the greater the risk for heart disease.

_____ 6. Bile acid sequestrants work by binding bile acids to form an insoluble substance that is excreted in the feces, causing the liver to use cholesterol to make more bile.

_____ 7. HMG-CoA reductase inhibitors are used to treat high serum triglyceride levels when diet alone has not lowered the level.

_____ 8. All fibric acid derivatives work in the same way.

_____ 9. The fibric acid derivatives may trigger the formation of gallstones or cholecystitis.

_____ 10. Niacin is used to help lower serum cholesterol levels.

VI. MULTIPLE CHOICE

Circle the letter of the best answer.

1. The target LDL level for treatment is _____.
   a. less than 130 mg/dL
   b. greater than 40 mg/dL
   c. between 150 and 200 mg/dL
   d. equal to the cholesterol level
   e. None of the above

2. Mr. H has had no decrease in his cholesterol level with a diet and exercise program. Which of the three types of antihyperlipidemic drugs might the health care provider recommend?
   a. Niacin
   b. Fibric acid derivatives
   c. HMG-CoA reductase inhibitors
   d. Bile acid sequestrants
   e. Any of the above

3. Bile acid sequestrants _____.
   a. should be administered apart from other medications
   b. decrease the absorption of other drugs
   c. are contraindicated in complete biliary obstruction
   d. may increase the risk of bleeding when given with oral anticoagulants
   e. All of the above

4. _____ appears to inhibit the manufacture of cholesterol or promote the breakdown of cholesterol.
   a. Niacin
   b. Bile acid sequestrants
   c. HMG-CoA reductase inhibitors
   d. Fibric acid derivatives
   e. All of the above

5. Mrs. S is being treated with pravastatin. At her regular check-up she reports that she has just started to note muscle pain and has had a low-grade fever. As part of her health care team, you tell her _____.
   a. that she probably has a touch of the flu
   b. it is a common adverse reaction of her medicine
   c. it will go away as she gets used to the medicine
   d. that you will report this to her health care provider immediately
   e. it means that the medication is working

6. Which fibric acid derivative is not thought to be effective for the prevention of coronary heart disease?
   a. clofibrate
   b. gemfibrozil
   c. fenofibrate
   d. niacin
   e. Both a and b

7. Mrs. L wants to know why so many people take garlic as a dietary supplement to help their cardiovascular system. As a health care worker you can explain to her that garlic _____.
   a. helps to lower serum cholesterol and triglyceride levels
   b. improves the HDL to LDL ratio
   c. lowers blood pressure
   d. helps prevent atherosclerosis
   e. All of the above

8. Ms. M has been faithfully taking her antihyperlipidemic drug for almost 4 months with no improvement in her blood cholesterol levels. What treatment options are left for her with medications?
   a. She should continue with the same therapy for 3 more months
   b. Her drug regimen may need to be modified
   c. She should discontinue all of her drugs because they obviously are not working
   d. She may need multiple medications
   e. She may need higher doses of her current drug

VII. RECALL FACTS

Indicate which of the following statements are facts with an F. If the statement is not a fact, leave the line blank.

ABOUT BILE ACID SEQUESTRANT ADMINISTRATION

____ 1. Should be taken before meals unless instructed otherwise

____ 2. Cholestyramine powder can be placed safely on the tongue.

____ 3. Colestipol granules do not dissolve, so the preparation must be stirred until it is ready to drink.

____ 4. Colesevelam tablets can be taken without regard for meals.

____ 5. It is uncommon to experience constipation, flatulence, nausea, or heartburn after administration of bile acid sequestrants.

ABOUT RISK FACTORS FOR DEVELOPING HYPERLIPIDEMIA

____ 1. Cigarette smoking

____ 2. Hypertension

____ 3. Obesity

____ 4. Anemia

____ 5. Diabetes

____ 6. Age

VIII. FILL IN THE BLANKS

Fill in the blanks using words from the list below.

LDLs	garlic	niacin	constipation
HDLs	240	150	rhabdomyolysis

1. A cholesterol level greater than _____ mg/dL and a triglyceride level greater than _____ mg/dL could contribute to atherosclerosis.

2. _____ transport cholesterol to peripheral cells while _____ carry cholesterol from the peripheral cells to the liver to be metabolized.

3. A common adverse reaction of bile acid sequestrants is _____.

4. _____ is a rare but serious adverse reaction of HMG-CoA reductase inhibitors.

5. Some adverse reactions of _____ include flushing of the skin, a sensation of warmth, and severe itching or tingling.

6. _____ is excreted in breast milk and may cause colic in infants.

IX. LIST

List the requested number of items.

1. List four factors that contribute to hyperlipidemia.

   a. _____

   b. _____

   c. _____

   d. _____

2. List four therapeutic life changes that can help lower a patient's cholesterol level.

   a. _____

   b. _____

   c. _____

   d. _____

3. List four things that a patient may do to lessen constipation that results from bile acid sequestrant use.

   a. _____

   b. _____

   c. _____

   d. _____

4. List the two types of antihyperlipidemic drugs that may lead to rhabdomyolysis.

   a. _____

   b. _____

5. List four things that a health care provider should do when dealing with a patient using diet and drugs to control high blood cholesterol levels.

   a. _____

   b. _____

   c. _____

   d. _____

X. CLINICAL APPLICATIONS

1. Mrs. Z is taking a bile acid sequestrant to help lower her serum cholesterol level. What adverse reactions might she expect while taking this medication?

XI. CASE STUDY

Mr. X. has been put on an HMG-CoA reductase inhibitor medication to lower his cholesterol. The health care staff is planning activities for him which will assist in the understanding of hyperlipidemia management.

1. Activities which may be recommended for Mr. X. include all of the following except

   a. referral to a dietician.
   b. a dietary teaching session.
   c. a hospital lecture about diet restrictions.
   d. a French cooking class.

2. The health care provider should do the following when using diet and drugs to control high blood cholesterol

   a. provide a written copy of the dietary plan and review its contents.
   b. emphasize that drug therapy alone will not significantly lower blood cholesterol levels.
   c. reinforce the importance of adhering to the prescribed diet.
   d. All of the above

3. Mr. X. is taking an HMG-CoA reductase inhibitor. Which of the following signs or symptoms should the health care provider be made aware of?

   a. Nausea
   b. Muscle pain
   c. Extreme fatigue
   d. Muscle tenderness
   e. All of the above

23

Anticoagulant and Thrombolytic Drugs

I. MATCH THE FOLLOWING

Match the term from Column A with the correct definition from Column B.

COLUMN A

___ 1. Thrombolytic drugs

___ 2. Hemostasis

___ 3. Prothrombin

___ 4. Fibrinolytic drugs

___ 5. Thrombosis

___ 6. Thrombus

COLUMN B

A. The formation of a clot

B. Blood clot

C. Drugs designed to dissolve existing clots

D. A substance that is essential for the clotting of blood

E. A process that stops bleeding in a blood vessel

F. Another name for thrombolytic drugs

II. MATCH THE FOLLOWING

Match the type of anticoagulant or anticoagulant antagonist from Column A with the drug name from Column B. You may use an answer more than once.

COLUMN A

___ 1. enoxaparin sodium

___ 2. heparin

___ 3. protamine sulfate

___ 4. anisindione

___ 5. warfarin sodium

___ 6. danaparoid sodium

___ 7. dalteparin sodium

___ 8. tinzaparin sodium

___ 9. phytonadione

COLUMN B

A. Coumadin

B. Indandione derivative

C. Unfractionated heparin

D. Fractionated heparin

E. Anticoagulant antagonist

III. MATCH THE FOLLOWING

Match the generic anticoagulant or thrombolytic from Column A with the trade name from Column B.

COLUMN A

_____ 1. anisindione

_____ 2. dalteparin sodium

_____ 3. urokinase

_____ 4. danaparoid sodium

_____ 5. alteplase

_____ 6. enoxaparin sodium

_____ 7. tinzaparin sodium

_____ 8. streptokinase

_____ 9. warfarin sodium

_____ 10. phytonadione

COLUMN B

A. Coumadin

B. Lovenox

C. Innohep

D. Fragmin

E. Aqua-MEPHYTON

F. Orgaran

G. Activase

H. Abbokinase

I. Miradon

J. Streptase

IV. TRUE OR FALSE

Indicate whether each statement is True (T) or False (F).

_____ 1. Anticoagulant therapy can prevent clots from forming.

_____ 2. Thrombolytic drugs can prevent the formation of a thrombus.

_____ 3. The most common adverse reaction of warfarin sodium is bleeding.

_____ 4. Warfarin sodium overdoses may be treated by administering vitamin K.

_____ 5. Warfarin sodium may safely be used during pregnancy and lactation.

_____ 6. Heparin is not a single drug.

_____ 7. Clotting is the chief complication of heparin administration.

_____ 8. LMWHs cause fewer adverse reactions than heparin.

_____ 9. Protamine sulfate counteracts the effects of heparin.

_____ 10. Heparin must be given through the parenteral route.

_____ 11. LMWHs are given only in the hospital, but heparin can be administered at home.

_____ 12. Thrombolytics dissolve certain types of blood clots and can reopen vessels after they have been occluded.

_____ 13. The most common adverse reaction caused by thrombolytic drug use is bleeding.

V. MULTIPLE CHOICE

Circle the letter of the best answer.

1. Anticoagulants _____.
   a. have no direct effect on an existing thrombus
   b. do not reverse any damage from a thrombus
   c. can prevent additional clots from forming
   d. are sometimes called blood thinners
   e. All of the above

2. All of the following drugs are anticoagulants except _____.
   a. warfarin sodium
   b. streptokinase
   c. anisindione

   d. fractionated heparin (LMWH)
   e. unfractionated heparin (heparin sodium)

3. Warfarin sodium _____.
   a. interferes with the production of vitamin K-dependent clotting factors
   b. works better if given with vitamin C
   c. prevents the formation of erythropoietin by the kidneys
   d. is contraindicated in patients with iron deficiency anemia
   e. can produce a decrease in the effectiveness of leucovorin calcium

4. Mr. S is currently taking warfarin sodium. His last PT and INR were within the therapeutic range. He called his health care provider's office this afternoon saying that his gums are still bleeding after brushing his teeth this morning. As the health care worker who took the call you should _____.

   a. tell him to buy a soft toothbrush
   b. tell him not to worry, this is normal
   c. tell him not to brush his teeth
   d. report this immediately to the health care provider
   e. tell him to call back in a few days if he continues to bleed

5. Diet can influence the effectiveness of warfarin sodium therapy. It is best for patients taking warfarin sodium to _____.

   a. eat a diet high in vitamin K
   b. eat a diet low in vitamin K
   c. eat a diet with a consistent amount of vitamin K
   d. totally eliminate vitamin K from their diet
   e. change to injection-administered warfarin sodium

6. All of the following are true regarding heparin except what?

   a. Heparin may be given orally.
   b. Heparin inhibits the formation of fibrin clots.
   c. Heparin inhibits the conversion of fibrinogen to fibrin.
   d. Heparin has no effects on existing clots.
   e. Heparin inactivates several factors needed for clotting.

7. Heparin administration can cause bleeding that _____.

   a. can be at any site
   b. is more common in individuals older than 60
   c. is more common in women
   d. should be reported immediately to the health care provider
   e. All of the above

8. LMWHs are contraindicated in all of the following patients except _____.

   a. those with a known hypersensitivity to the drug or heparin
   b. those with deep vein thrombosis
   c. those with a known hypersensitivity to pork products
   d. those with thrombocytopenia
   e. those with active bleeding

9. All of the following will increase the effects of heparin when administered together except _____.

   a. NSAIDs
   b. aspirin
   c. penicillin
   d. protamine sulfate
   e. cephalosporin

10. Thrombolytic drugs work by _____.

    a. breaking down prothrombin
    b. converting plasminogen to plasmin
    c. forming fibrin clots
    d. converting prothrombin to thrombin
    e. None of the above

11. Patients being treated with thrombolytic drugs _____.

    a. should not be given an anticoagulant
    b. cannot have had recent intracranial surgery
    c. should be physically active
    d. should be monitored for signs of bleeding and hemorrhage
    e. Both b and d

12. Thrombolytic drugs work best to dissolve thrombi when they are _____.

    a. given as soon as possible after the formation of a thrombus
    b. given within 4 to 6 hours after the formation of a thrombus
    c. given within 24 hours after the formation of a thrombus
    d. given in conjunction with protamine sulfate
    e. injected directly into the thrombus

VI. RECALL FACTS

Indicate which of the following statements are facts with an F. If the statement is not a fact, leave the line blank.

ABOUT MEDICATIONS THAT MAY CAUSE AN INCREASE IN THE EFFECT OF WARFARIN SODIUM

____ 1. Oral contraceptives
____ 2. Acetaminophen
____ 3. Ascorbic acid
____ 4. Barbiturates
____ 5. Beta blockers
____ 6. Diuretics
____ 7. Aminoglycosides
____ 8. Tetracycline
____ 9. Vitamin K
____ 10. NSAIDs
____ 11. Cephalosporins
____ 12. Loop diuretics

ABOUT SITUATIONS IN WHICH HEPARIN IS USED

____ 1. Atrial fibrillation with embolus formation

____ 2. Prevention of clotting in medical equipment

____ 3. Treatment of DIC

____ 4. Labor and delivery

____ 5. Prevention of clotting in arterial and heart surgery

____ 6. Destruction of clots already formed

VII. FILL IN THE BLANKS

Fill in the blanks using words from the list below.

clot formation	PT	APTT	10	4
1	increase	decrease	bleeding	6

1. The health care provider should be notified immediately if a patient taking warfarin sodium has evidence of _____.

2. Vitamin K administration will enhance _____ and return the PT to an acceptable level in approximately _____ hours.

3. A significant _____ in blood pressure or a(n) _____ in pulse rate may indicate internal bleeding.

4. The laboratory test used to manage warfarin sodium therapy is the _____, whereas the _____ test is used to monitor heparin therapy.

5. Heparin causes anticoagulation after _____ dose, with maximum effects within _____ minutes, but the clotting time will return to normal within _____ hours unless additional doses are given.

VIII. LIST

List the requested number of items.

1. List five uses of warfarin sodium.

   a. _____

   b. _____

   c. _____

   d. _____

   e. _____

2. List four symptoms of warfarin sodium overdosage.

   a. _____

   b. _____

   c. _____

   d. _____

3. List six common cooking herbs warfarin sodium that should not be combined with because of the additive effects and increased risk of bleeding.

   a. _____

   b. _____

   c. _____

   d. _____

   e. _____

   f. _____

4. List six conditions in which heparin therapy is contraindicated.

    a. _____

    b. _____

    c. _____

    d. _____

    e. _____

    f. _____

5. List the four uses of thrombolytic drugs.

    a. _____

    b. _____

    c. _____

    d. _____

IX. CLINICAL APPLICATIONS

1. Mrs. G was hospitalized with deep vein thrombosis 2 weeks ago and was sent home with a prescription for warfarin sodium. Her current INR is 2.7. What information should Mrs. G be aware of while taking warfarin sodium?

X. CASE STUDY

Mr. K., age 61, is experiencing a myocardial infarction. He has been taken to a rural hospital that is 250 miles from a cardiac catheterization laboratory. His physician has decided to administer a thrombolytic agent to open his blocked coronary artery.

1. Before the medication is given, Mr. K.'s health history is obtained. What conditions would make a thrombolytic agent contraindicated?

    a. Active bleeding
    b. History of stroke
    c. Aneurysm
    d. Recent intracranial surgery
    e. All of the above

2. Mr. K. is given the thrombolytic drug along with heparin. What is the purpose of giving heparin?

    a. To help dissolve the existing clot
    b. To reverse the effects of the thrombolytic
    c. To prevent another thrombus from forming
    d. None of the above

3. While he receives the thrombolytic drug, Mr. K. is continually assessed for an anaphylactic reaction. Symptoms of this would be

    a. difficulty breathing.
    b. wheezing.
    c. hives.
    d. All of the above

24

Antianemia Drugs

I. MATCH THE FOLLOWING

Match the generic drug name from Column A with the type of anemia it is used to treat from Column B. You may use an answer more than once.

COLUMN A

_____ 1. ferrous sulfate

_____ 2. epoetin alfa

_____ 3. folic acid

_____ 4. iron sucrose

_____ 5. sodium ferric gluconate

_____ 6. vitamin B_{12}

_____ 7. darbepoetin alfa

_____ 8. ferrous fumarate

COLUMN B

A. Anemia associated with chronic renal failure

B. Iron deficiency anemia

C. Megaloblastic anemia

D. B_{12} deficiency

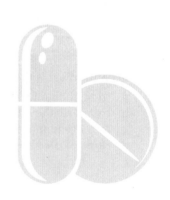

II. MATCH THE FOLLOWING

Match the generic drug name from Column A with the trade name from Column B.

COLUMN A

_____ 1. darbepoetin alfa

_____ 2. ferrous fumarate

_____ 3. epoetin alfa

_____ 4. ferrous sulfate

_____ 5. vitamin B_{12}

_____ 6. ferrous gluconate

_____ 7. folic acid

_____ 8. sodium ferric gluconate

_____ 9. iron dextran

COLUMN B

A. Epogen

B. Fergon

C. Feosol

D. Aranesp

E. Femiron

F. Folvite

G. Venofer

H. Calomist

I. Ferrlecit

III. TRUE OR FALSE

Indicate whether each statement is True (T) or False (F).

_____ 1. Iron preparations act by depleting iron stores.

_____ 2. An adverse reaction of oral iron preparations is constipation.

_____ 3. Hypersensitivity reactions have never been reported with the use of parenteral iron.

_____ 4. Patients with uncontrolled hypertension should not be prescribed either epoetin alfa or darbepoetin alfa.

_____ 5. Leucovorin calcium increases the effectiveness of anticonvulsants.

_____ 6. Vitamin B_{12} therapy is contraindicated in patients allergic to cobalt.

IV. MULTIPLE CHOICE

Circle the letter of the best answer.

1. Which parenteral iron preparation is used for the treatment of iron deficiency anemia when oral treatments cannot be used because of gastrointestinal intolerance?

   a. ferrous sulfate
   b. iron dextran
   c. ferrous gluconate
   d. ferrous fumarate
   e. iron sucrose

2. Iron compounds are contraindicated in which of the following patients?

   a. Patients with any anemia except iron deficiency anemia
   b. Patients with a known hypersensitivity to the drug
   c. Patients with sulfate sensitivity
   d. Patients with cardiovascular disease
   e. Both a and b

3. Epoetin alfa is used to treat _____.

   a. anemia caused by chemotherapy
   b. anemia of chronic renal failure

   c. anemia in patients undergoing elective nonvascular surgery
   d. Both a and c
   e. Answers a, b, and c

4. Darbepoetin _____.

   a. acts by stimulating erythropoiesis
   b. elevates or maintains RBC levels
   c. decreases the need for transfusions
   d. can be used to treat anemia caused by chronic renal failure
   e. All of the above

5. All of the following are correct regarding leucovorin calcium except that it _____.

   a. uses a derivative of folic acid
   b. can be administered orally or parenterally
   c. can be used to rescue normal cells from methotrexate
   d. it can be used safely in patients with pernicious anemia
   e. has few adverse reactions

V. RECALL FACTS

Indicate which of the following statements are facts with an F. If the statement is not a fact, leave the line blank.

ABOUT PATIENT INSTRUCTIONS FOR TAKING EPOETIN ALFA

_____ 1. Report any numbness or tingling of extremities

_____ 2. You may control joint pain with analgesics

_____ 3. Report any severe headaches, dyspnea, or chest pain

_____ 4. It is important to keep all appointments for blood testing

_____ 5. Avoid the use of multivitamin preparations unless they are approved by your health care provider.

VI. FILL IN THE BLANKS

Fill in the blanks using words from the list below.

increases   pernicious anemia   depleted   decrease
elevating   folinic acid   leucovorin rescue

1. Iron preparations act by _____ the serum iron concentration, which replenishes hemoglobin and _____ iron stores.

2. Ascorbic acid _____ the absorption of oral iron, whereas antacids _____ oral iron absorption.

3. _____ is a type of megaloblastic anemia that results from a deficiency of intrinsic factor.

4. _____ or _____ is the technique of administering leucovorin after a large dose of methotrexate to rescue normal cells and allow them to survive.

VII. LIST

List the requested number of items.

1. List four adverse reactions that when present while administering parenteral iron need to be reported to the health care provider.

   a. _____

   b. _____

   c. _____

   d. _____

2. List four types of patients in whom a vitamin B_{12} deficiency may be seen.

   a. _____

   b. _____

   c. _____

   d. _____

3. List four types of patients who may be treated with epoetin alfa.

   a. _____

   b. _____

   c. _____

   d. _____

VIII. CLINICAL APPLICATIONS

1. Mr. F has chronic renal failure and is undergoing dialysis twice weekly for this condition. Anemia has developed as a result of his kidneys failing to produce adequate amount of erythropoietins. Choose the best drug to treat Mr. F's anemia and explain the drug's action.

IX. CASE STUDY

Mr. J. has developed iron deficiency anemia. He has visited his health care provider and is being placed on an iron medication.

1. What drugs should he be told not to take while he is on iron unless he checks with his health care provider?

    a. Antacids
    b. Tetracycline
    c. Penicillamine
    d. Fluoroquinolones
    e. All of the above

2. What changes in bowel habit could he encounter?

    a. Darkening of the stools
    b. Constipation
    c. Stools are always normal
    d. Diarrhea
    e. Answers a, b, and d

3. How do iron preparations work?

    a. They elevate the serum iron concentration
    b. They replenish hemoglobin
    c. They "rescue" normal cells from the destruction caused by methotrexate
    d. Both a and b

DRUGS THAT AFFECT THE URINARY SYSTEM

VI

25

Diuretics

I. MATCH THE FOLLOWING

Match the term from Column A with the correct definition from Column B.

COLUMN A

____ 1. Diuretic
____ 2. Edema
____ 3. Hyperkalemia
____ 4. Hypokalemia

COLUMN B

A. High blood level of potassium
B. Retention of excess fluid
C. Low blood level of potassium
D. A drug that increases the secretion of urine by the kidneys

---

II. MATCH THE FOLLOWING

Match the generic diuretic from Column A with the correct trade name from Column B.

COLUMN A

____ 1. torsemide
____ 2. ethacrynic acid
____ 3. spironolactone
____ 4. triamterene
____ 5. mannitol
____ 6. amiloride
____ 7. furosemide
____ 8. metolazone
____ 9. chlorothiazide
____ 10. methazolamide

COLUMN B

A. Osmitrol
B. Zaroxolyn
C. Lasix
D. Edecrin
E. Demadex
F. Diuril
G. Midamor
H. Neptazane
I. Aldactone
J. Dyrenium

III. MATCH THE FOLLOWING

Match the trade name from Column A with the correct type of diuretic from Column B. You may use an answer more than once.

COLUMN A

_____ 1. Thalitone

_____ 2. Aldactone

_____ 3. Edecrin

_____ 4. Midamor

_____ 5. Diamox

_____ 6. Demadex

_____ 7. Microzide

_____ 8. Ureaphil

_____ 9. Zaroxolyn

_____ 10. Dyrenium

_____ 11. Neptazane

_____ 12. Osmitrol

COLUMN B

A. Carbonic anhydrase inhibitor

B. Loop diuretic

C. Osmotic diuretic

D. Potassium-sparing diuretic

E. Thiazides and related diuretics

IV. TRUE OR FALSE

Indicate whether each statement is True (T) or False (F).

_____ 1. Diuretics are only used to treat hypertension.

_____ 2. Carbonic anhydrase inhibitors can be used to treat glaucoma.

_____ 3. Adverse reactions associated with short-term therapy with carbonic anhydrase inhibitors are rare.

_____ 4. Loop diuretics work by increasing the excretion of sodium and chloride by stimulating their reabsorption in the proximal and distal tubules and in the loop of Henle.

_____ 5. Torsemide acts primarily in the ascending portion of the loop of Henle.

_____ 6. Bumetanide acts primarily on the proximal tubule of the nephron.

_____ 7. Patients with diabetes who take loop diuretics may experience a decrease in blood glucose levels.

_____ 8. A potential adverse reaction of loop diuretics is orthostatic hypertension.

_____ 9. It is safe to give infants ethacrynic acid.

_____ 10. A patient who is sensitive to the sulfonamides may have an allergic reaction to bumetanide.

_____ 11. Osmotic diuretics increase the density of the filtrate in the glomerulus.

_____ 12. Osmotic diuretics only allow water to be excreted.

_____ 13. Aldactone antagonizes the action of aldosterone.

_____ 14. Potassium-sparing diuretics may cause hyperkalemia in patients with inadequate fluid intake.

_____ 15. Older adults are more at risk for electrolyte imbalances while taking diuretics.

_____ 16. Cardiac arrest may occur when a patient taking a potassium preparation is administered a potassium-sparing diuretic.

_____ 17. Thiazides work by inhibiting the reabsorption of sodium and chloride ions.

_____ 18. The electrolyte and fluid loss associated with thiazide use can often be easily corrected.

_____ 19. Dandelion root is an effective natural diuretic.

_____ 20. The duration of activity of most diuretics is 8 hours or less.

_____ 21. The most common electrolyte imbalances experienced by patients taking a diuretic are the loss of potassium and water.

_____ 22. Older adults should be monitored for hypokalemia when taking a potassium-sparing diuretic.

_____ 23. Most herbal diuretics are either ineffective or no more effective than caffeine.

V. MULTIPLE CHOICE

Circle the letter of the best answer.

1. Carbonic anhydrase inhibitors work by _____.
   a. inhibiting the action of the enzyme carbonic anhydrase
   b. increasing the production of the enzyme carbonic anhydrase
   c. decreasing the production of the enzyme carbonic anhydrase
   d. stimulating the action of the enzyme carbonic anhydrase
   e. None of the above

2. Carbonic anhydrase inhibitors have the effect of excretion of _____ by the kidneys.
   a. sodium
   b. potassium
   c. bicarbonate
   d. water
   e. All of the above

3. _____, a carbonic anhydrase inhibitor, is used in the treatment of simple (open-angle) glaucoma and secondary glaucoma.
   a. Neptazane
   b. Diamox
   c. Bumex
   d. Ismotic
   e. Edecrin

4. All of the following, except one, are patients in whom carbonic anhydrase inhibitors would be contraindicated. Which is the exception?
   a. Patients with electrolyte imbalances
   b. Patients with severe kidney dysfunction
   c. Patients with asthma
   d. Patients with anuria
   e. Patients with liver dysfunction

5. The drug _____ is an example of a loop diuretic.
   a. furosemide
   b. acetazolamide
   c. ethacrynic acid
   d. Both a and c
   e. All of the above

6. The drug _____ can be used for the short-term management of ascites.
   a. furosemide
   b. torsemide
   c. bumetanide
   d. ethacrynic acid
   e. mannitol

7. Ototoxicity can occur if a loop diuretic is given with a _____.
   a. thrombolytic
   b. aminoglycoside
   c. cardiac drug
   d. NSAID
   e. lithium drug

8. Loop diuretics may increase the effectiveness of which of the following drugs?
   a. Thrombolytics
   b. Anticoagulants
   c. Propranolol
   d. Lithium
   e. All of the above

9. The drug _____ is an osmotic diuretic that is administered intravenously.
   a. urea
   b. glycerin
   c. mannitol
   d. isosorbide
   e. Both a and c

10. Triamterene is a(n) _____.
    a. osmotic diuretic
    b. potassium-sparing diuretic
    c. loop diuretic
    d. thiazide
    e. carbonic anhydrase inhibitor

11. Potassium-sparing diuretics are used to treat _____.
    a. chronic heart failure
    b. hypertension
    c. edema caused by chronic heart failure
    d. Both a and c
    e. All of the above

12. In which of the following patients are potassium-sparing diuretics contraindicated?
    a. Patients with hyperkalemia
    b. Patients with anuria
    c. Patients with significant renal impairment
    d. Patients with serious electrolyte imbalances
    e. All of the above

13. Administration of a thiazide will result in the
    _____.
    a. retention of potassium
    b. excretion of potassium
    c. excretion of sodium, chloride, and water
    d. retention of sodium, chloride, and water
    e. None of the above

14. Some thiazides contain _____, which may cause
    bronchial asthma in patients who are sensitive to
    the drug.
    a. tartrazine
    b. theophylline

    c. aminoglycosides
    d. penicillin
    e. glucose

15. Patients taking thiazides or related diuretics may
    experience _____ as an adverse reaction.
    a. azotemia
    b. gout
    c. hyperglycemia
    d. All of the above
    e. None of the above

VI. RECALL FACTS

Indicate which of the following statements are facts with an F. If the statement is not a fact, leave the line blank.

ABOUT THOSE INSTANCES IN WHICH CONCURRENT THIAZIDE ADMINISTRATION WILL INCREASE THE OTHER DRUG'S EFFECTS

____ 1. Allopurinol hypersensitivity

____ 2. Anticoagulant effects

____ 3. Antidiabetic drugs

____ 4. Anesthetics

____ 5. Uric acid levels

____ 6. Glycoside toxicity

VII. FILL IN THE BLANKS

Fill in the blanks using words from the list below.

renal dysfunction   mannitol   electrolyte imbalance   tubules   chloride   gynecomastia
cardiac arrhythmias   avoided   C   furosemide   increased   reabsorption
excretion   hypokalemia   hourly   sulfonamides   B

1. Most diuretics act on the _____ of
   the kidney nephron.

2. Diuretics are Pregnancy Category _____
   and _____ drugs.

3. Patients taking carbonic anhydrase inhibitors have
   a(n) _____ risk of cyclosporine
   toxicity when the drug is administered with
   acetazolamide.

4. Bumetanide primarily increases the excretion of
   _____.

5. _____ is the drug of choice when
   rapid diuresis is needed.

6. Loop diuretics are used cautiously in patients with
   _____.

7. When administered to a patient in a fasting
   state, osmotic diuretics may result in a rapid
   _____.

8. _____ is contraindicated in
   patients with active intracranial bleeding.

9. Midamor acts by depressing the
   _____ of sodium and by
   depressing the _____ of potassium.

10. _____ may occur in patients taking
    spironolactone.

11. A cross-sensitivity reaction may occur with thia-
    zides and _____.

12. Mannitol requires _____
    monitoring of urine output.

13. In patients with edema who are being treated with a diuretic, a weight loss of approximately _____ per day is desirable.

14. An older adult is monitored for _____ if taking a loop or a thiazide diuretic.

15. Patients concurrently receiving a diuretic and a digitalis glycoside require frequent monitoring for _____.

16. Diuretic teas should be _____.

VIII. LIST

List the requested number of items.

1. List the five types of diuretic drugs.

   a. _____

   b. _____

   c. _____

   d. _____

   e. _____

2. List five adverse reactions caused by long-term use of carbonic anhydrase inhibitors.

   a. _____

   b. _____

   c. _____

   d. _____

   e. _____

3. List three uses of loop diuretics.

   a. _____

   b. _____

   c. _____

4. List three uses of osmotic diuretics.

   a. _____

   b. _____

   c. _____

5. List the three trade names of osmotic diuretic drugs.

   a. _____

   b. _____

   c. _____

6. List five types of patients in whom hyperkalemia may occur when treated with a potassium-sparing diuretic.

   a. _____

   b. _____

   c. _____

   d. _____

   e. _____

7. List two uses of thiazides.

   a. _____

   b. _____

8. List five symptoms of hyperkalemia.

   a. _____

   b. _____

   c. _____

   d. _____

   e. _____

9. List five warning signs of fluid and electrolyte imbalance.

   a. _____

   b. _____

   c. _____

   d. _____

   e. _____

10. List five herbal diuretics.

   a. _____

   b. _____

   c. _____

   d. _____

   e. _____

IX. CLINICAL APPLICATIONS

1. Mrs. K, age 63, has been diagnosed with chronic heart failure. As a result of this condition, she has edema, which must be treated immediately. Using your text as a guide, answer the following questions.

   a. Which type of diuretic would most likely be chosen to treat Mrs. K's edema?

   b. Which specific drug is the drug of choice when rapid diuresis is required?

   c. What are the most common adverse reaction associated with this type of diuretic?

X. CASE STUDY

Mr. Jones, an 80-year-old retired college professor, has been diagnosed with hypertension. His physician has decided to put him on a potassium-sparing diuretic.

1. What condition is Mr. Jones most at risk for while on this medication?

   a. Hypokalemia
   b. Hyperkalemia
   c. Hypermagnesemia
   d. Orthostatic hypotension

2. What are the symptoms that Mr. Jones may experience if this occurs?

   a. Paresthesia
   b. Muscular weakness
   c. Fatigue
   d. Bradycardia
   e. All of the above

3. Spironolactone was prescribed for Mr. Jones. Which of the following describe the action of this drug.

   a. It antagonizes the action of aldosterone.
   b. It enhances the action of aldosterone.
   c. It causes sodium, potassium, and water to be excreted.
   d. It causes sodium and water to be excreted.
   e. Both a and d

26

Urinary Anti-Infectives

I. MATCH THE FOLLOWING

Match the term from Column A with the correct definition from Column B.

COLUMN A

_____ 1. Dysuria

_____ 2. Urinary frequency

_____ 3. Urinary urgency

_____ 4. Bacteriostatic

_____ 5. Bactericidal

_____ 6. Creatinine clearance

_____ 7. Cystitis

_____ 8. Anti-infective

_____ 9. Urinary tract infection

COLUMN B

A. Painful or difficult urination

B. Frequent urination day and night

C. Strong, sudden need to urinate

D. Destroys bacteria

E. Slows or retards the multiplication of bacteria

F. Urinary tract infection of the bladder

G. The rate at which creatinine is excreted from the urine over time

H. A drug used to treat infection

I. An infection caused by pathogenic microorganisms of one or more structures of the urinary tract

II. MATCH THE FOLLOWING

Match the generic drug name from Column A with the correct trade name from Column B.

COLUMN A

_____ 1. doripenem

_____ 2. fosfomycin

_____ 3. methenamine hippurate

_____ 4. nitrofurantoin

_____ 5. trimethoprim (TMP)

_____ 6. trimethoprim and sulfamethoxazole (TMP-SMZ)

COLUMN B

A. Doribax

B. Bactrim

C. Hiprex

D. Macrobid

E. Primsol

F. Monurol

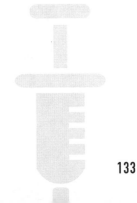

133

III. MATCH THE FOLLOWING

Match the drug trade name from Column A with the type of drug from Column B. You may use an answer more than once.

COLUMN A

_____ 1. Doribax

_____ 2. Hiprex

_____ 3. Macrobid

_____ 4. Primsol

_____ 5. Bactrim

_____ 6. Monurol

COLUMN B

A. Anti-infective drug; single ingredient

B. Urinary anti-infective combination drug

IV. TRUE OR FALSE

Indicate whether each statement is True (T) or False (F).

_____ 1. Urinary anti-infectives that are taken by the oral or parenteral route do not achieve significant levels in the bloodstream.

_____ 2. Ammonia and formaldehyde formed from the breakdown of methenamine and methenamine salts are bactericidal.

_____ 3. Nitrofurantoin may be bacteriostatic or bactericidal.

_____ 4. Fosfomycin is bactericidal.

_____ 5. Pulmonary reactions have been reported with the use of nitrofurantoin.

_____ 6. No serious drug interactions have been reported with methenamine.

V. MULTIPLE CHOICE

Circle the letter of the best answer.

1. Large doses of methenamine may result in _____.
   a. cystitis
   b. bladder irritation
   c. burning on urination
   d. Answers a and b
   e. Answers b and c

2. Fosfomycin acts by _____.
   a. lysing the bacterial cell wall
   b. interfering with the metabolism of dextrose
   c. interrupting RNA replication
   d. interfering with cell wall synthesis
   e. Answers a and c

3. Nausea can be an adverse reaction to _____.
   a. nitrofurantoin
   b. fosfomycin
   c. doripenem
   d. methenamine
   e. All of the above

4. Nitrofurantoin may cause a(n) _____ which needs to be reported to the health care provider and the next dose is not taken until the patient is evaluated.
   a. blood glucose elevation
   b. severe arrhythmia
   c. permanent visual disturbance
   d. pulmonary reaction
   e. ototoxicity reaction

5. Cranberries _____.
   a. inhibit bacteria from attaching to the walls of the urinary tract
   b. have no known adverse reactions
   c. have no known drug interactions
   d. All of the above

VI. FILL IN THE BLANKS

Fill in the blanks using words from the list below.

methenamine   urine   antacids   trimethoprim   megaloblastic anemia   urinary tract

1. Urinary anti-infective drugs exert their major anti-bacterial effects in the _____.

2. _____ breaks down to form ammonia and formaldehyde.

3. Nitrofurantoin's mode of action is dependent on the concentration of the drug in the _____.

4. _____ acts by interfering with the metabolism of folinic acid by the bacteria.

5. When taking methenamine the patient should not use _____ containing sodium bicarbonate or sodium carbonate.

6. Trimethoprim is used with caution in patients with _____ caused by folate deficiency.

VII. LIST

List the requested number of items.

1. List five trade names of urinary anti-infective drugs.

   a. _____

   b. _____

   c. _____

   d. _____

   e. _____

2. List four adverse reactions associated with trimethoprim.

   a. _____

   b. _____

   c. _____

   d. _____

VIII. CLINICAL APPLICATIONS

1. Miss P was told that drinking a glass of cranberry juice everyday will cure her urinary tract infection. Explain to Miss P the role that cranberry juice can play in the treatment of her infection.

IX. CASE STUDY

Mr. G. has a urinary tract infection. His health care provider has prescribed nitrofurantoin for him. You are providing information to him about the drug before he leaves the clinic.

1. Nitrofurantoin must be taken _____.

   a. before meals
   b. with food or milk
   c. with orange juice
   d. any time of the day.

2. Adverse reactions to nitrofurantoin may include _____.

   a. nausea
   b. headache
   c. flatulence
   d. rash
   e. All of the above

3. Nitrofurantoin is contraindicated in _____.

   a. patients with kidney disease
   b. those with hypersensitivity to the drug
   c. lactating women
   d. All of the above

27

Miscellaneous Urinary Drugs

I. MATCH THE FOLLOWING

Match the term from Column A with the correct definition from Column B.

COLUMN A

____ 1. Dysuria

____ 2. Neurogenic bladder

____ 3. Overactive bladder

____ 4. Urge incontinence

____ 5. Nocturia

____ 6. Urinary urgency

COLUMN B

A. Painful or difficult urination

B. Excessive urination during the night

C. Strong, sudden need to urinate

D. Involuntary contractions of the detrusor or bladder muscle

E. Altered bladder function caused by a nervous system abnormality

F. Accidental loss of urine caused by a sudden and unstoppable need to urinate.

II. MATCH THE FOLLOWING

Match the generic drug name from Column A with the correct trade name from Column B.

COLUMN A

____ 1. fesoterodine

____ 2. darifenacin

____ 3. solifenacin

____ 4. phenazopyridine

____ 5. oxybutynin

____ 6. trospium

____ 7. tolterodine

COLUMN B

A. Toviaz

B. VESIcare

C. Detrol

D. Enablex

E. Ditropan

F. Sanctura

G. Pyridium

III. TRUE OR FALSE

Indicate whether each statement is True (T) or False (F).

____ 1. Flavoxate causes contraction of the detrusor muscle through action at the sympathetic receptors of the bladder.

____ 2. Flavoxate can cause mental confusion.

____ 3. Pyridium is a dye that has no anti-infective activity.

____ 4. Detrol is used to treat symptoms of overactive bladder.

____ 5. Phenazopyridine causes permanent reddish-orange discoloration of the urine.

IV. MULTIPLE CHOICE

Circle the letter of the best answer.

1. Which of the following is not considered to be an adverse reaction of tolterodine tartrate?

    a. Dry mouth
    b. Vertigo
    c. Dizziness
    d. Abdominal pain
    e. Perianal burning

2. Phenazopyridine appears to act by ____.

    a. interrupting bacterial RNA replication
    b. exerting a topical analgesic effect on the lining of the urinary tract
    c. interfering with bacterial multiplication
    d. inhibiting the metabolism of glucose
    e. None of the above

3. ____ is used to treat bladder instability caused by a neurogenic bladder.

    a. Pyridium
    b. Ditropan
    c. Detrol
    d. Enablex
    e. Toviaz

4. The drug ____ is an anticholinergic drug that inhibits bladder contractions.

    a. tolterodine
    b. phenazopyridine
    c. oxybutynin
    d. flavoxate
    e. fesoterodine

5. The drug ____ is contraindicated in patients with gastric blockage, abdominal bleeding, or urinary tract blockage.

    a. oxybutynin
    b. flavoxate
    c. darifenacin
    d. festoterodine
    e. All of the above

6. When haloperidol is administered with ____, there is an increased risk of tardive dyskinesia.

    a. oxybutynin
    b. flavoxate
    c. phenazopyridine
    d. darifenacin
    e. solifenacin

V. FILL IN THE BLANKS

Fill in the blanks using words from the list below.

analgesic   overactive bladder   liver disease   red–orange   dry mouth   neurogenic bladder

1. Phenazopyridine is a urinary _____ drug.

2. The most common adverse reaction of tolterodine is _____.

3. Darifenacin is used for _____.

4. Oxybutynin is used cautiously in patients with _____.

5. _____ is altered bladder function caused by a nervous system abnormality.

6. Phenazopyridine may cause a _____ discoloration of the urine.

VI. LIST

List the requested number of items.

1. List six conditions that flavoxate HCl is used to treat.

   a. _____

   b. _____

   c. _____

   d. _____

   e. _____

   f. _____

2. List four conditions in which oxybutynin should be used with caution.

   a. _____

   b. _____

   c. _____

   d. _____

VII. CLINICAL APPLICATIONS

1. Mr. C. has been put on an anticholinergic drug, tolterodine, for an overactive bladder. What are key points about this drug that he and his famivzly members should be told?

VIII. CASE STUDY

Mr. X. has been diagnosed with neurogenic bladder related to a spinal cord tumor. His physician has prescribed oxybutynin for this. Mr. X. lives in Florida.

1. Mr. X. needs to take appropriate precautions to avoid _____ because he lives in a hot climate.

   a. constipation
   b. urticaria
   c. heat prostration
   d. dry mouth

2. Which of the following is true about heat prostration?

   a. Fever is a symptom.
   b. Heat stroke is a symptom.
   c. Heat prostration is caused by decreased sweating.
   d. All of the above.

3. Oxybutynin is contraindicated in _____.

   a. glaucoma
   b. blockage of the gastrointestinal tract
   c. myasthenia gravis
   d. stroke
   e. Answers a, b, and c

VII

DRUGS THAT AFFECT THE GASTROINTESTINAL SYSTEM

28

Drugs That Affect the Stomach and Pancreas

I. MATCH THE FOLLOWING

Match the term from Column A with the correct definition from Column B.

COLUMN A

___ 1. Emetic

___ 2. Gastric stasis

___ 3. Hypersecretory

___ 4. Paralytic ileus

___ 5. Proton pump inhibitors

COLUMN B

A. Failure to move food normally out of the stomach

B. Excessive gastric secretion of hydrochloric acid

C. A drug that induces vomiting

D. Drugs with antisecretory properties

E. Lack of peristalsis or movement of the intestines

II. MATCH THE FOLLOWING

Match the generic proton pump inhibitor or miscellaneous gastrointestinal drug from Column A with the correct trade name from Column B.

COLUMN A

___ 1. sucralfate

___ 2. omeprazole

___ 3. rabeprazole

___ 4. esomeprazole

___ 5. misoprostol

___ 6. lansoprazole

COLUMN B

A. Prilosec

B. Aciphex

C. Prevacid

D. Carafate

E. Cytotec

F. Nexium

III. MATCH THE FOLLOWING

Match the generic antacid or anticholinergic drug name from Column A with the correct trade name from Column B.

COLUMN A

_____ 1. calcium carbonate

_____ 2. mepenzolate

_____ 3. glycopyrrolate

_____ 4. hyoscyamine sulfate

_____ 5. methscopolamine

_____ 6. metoclopramide

_____ 7. aluminum hydroxide

_____ 8. magnesium oxide

_____ 9. magnesium hydroxide

COLUMN B

A. Reglan

B. Alka-Mints

C. Pamine

D. Milk of Magnesia

E. Alternagel

F. Cantil

G. Anaspaz

H. Robinul

I. Mag-200

IV. MATCH THE FOLLOWING

Match the generic digestive enzyme, histamine H_2 antagonist, or antiflatulent drug from Column A with the correct trade name from Column B.

COLUMN A

_____ 1. famotidine

_____ 2. simethicone

_____ 3. pancrelipase

_____ 4. ranitidine

_____ 5. nizatidine

_____ 6. alpha-D-galactosidase

_____ 7. cimetidine

COLUMN B

A. Zantac

B. Gas-X

C. Tagamet

D. Beano

E. Pepcid

F. Creon

G. Axid

V. MATCH THE FOLLOWING

Match the trade name from Column A with the correct type of drug from Column B. You may use an answer more than once.

COLUMN A

_____ 1. Reglan

_____ 2. Pamine

_____ 3. Prevacid

_____ 4. Ipecac syrup

_____ 5. Robinul

_____ 6. Tagamet

_____ 7. Nexium

_____ 8. Pepcid

_____ 9. Prilosec

_____ 10. Creon

_____ 11. Tums

_____ 12. Mylicon

COLUMN B

A. Proton pump inhibitor

B. Antacid

C. Anticholinergic

D. Gastrointestinal stimulant

E. Histamine H_2 antagonist

F. Antiflatulent

G. Digestive enzyme

H. Emetic

VI. MATCH THE FOLLOWING

Match the miscellaneous gastrointestinal drug from Column A with the correct drug action from Column B.

COLUMN A	COLUMN B
____ 1. Misoprostol	A. Disrupts the integrity of bacterial cell wall
____ 2. Sucralfate	B. Local action on lining of the stomach
____ 3. Bismuth subsalicylate	C. Inhibits gastric acid secretion and increases mucus production

VII. TRUE OR FALSE

Indicate whether each statement is True (T) or False (F).

____ 1. Antacids work by changing the hydrochloric acid in the stomach to a base.

____ 2. Antacids can be used to treat other conditions not related to an acidic stomach.

____ 3. Oral iron products have a decreased pharmacological effect when administered with an antacid.

____ 4. Anticholinergics reduce gastric motility.

____ 5. Histamine H$_2$ antagonists have more adverse reactions than anticholinergic drugs when used to treat peptic ulcers.

____ 6. Reglan and Ilopan decrease the strength of spontaneous movement of the upper gastrointestinal tract and are used in the treatment of diarrhea.

____ 7. Ipecac should be given for all oral poisonings.

____ 8. Gastrointestinal stimulants are secreted in breast milk.

____ 9. Tardive dyskinesia as a result of gastrointestinal stimulant therapy is reversible.

____ 10. When Tagamet is given concurrently with morphine, the patient has an increased risk of respiratory depression.

____ 11. Motofen increases intestinal peristalsis.

____ 12. Charcoal works as an antiflatulent by reducing the amount of intestinal gas.

____ 13. Many adverse reactions have been reported by patients who have received an antiflatulent.

____ 14. Simethicone has no known drug interactions.

____ 15. Digestive enzymes are prescribed for patients with an overactive pancreas.

____ 16. Patients with acute pancreatitis should be prescribed high doses of digestive enzymes.

____ 17. Proton pump inhibitors work by suppressing gastric acid secretion.

____ 18. Bismuth subsalicylate can cause salicylate toxicity if used for an extended period.

____ 19. Chamomile is safe for all patients to take when the oral form is used.

VIII. MULTIPLE CHOICE

Circle the letter of the best answer.

1. In which of the following conditions are antacids used as part of the treatment regimen?

   a. Acid indigestion
   b. Sour stomach
   c. Peptic ulcer
   d. Heartburn
   e. All of the above

2. An antacid that contains magnesium may produce ____ as an adverse reaction.

   a. constipation
   b. anorexia
   c. dehydration
   d. metabolic alkalosis
   e. renal calculi

3. A calcium-containing antacid may produce ____ as an adverse reaction.

   a. rebound hypersecretion
   b. neurologic impairment
   c. severe diarrhea
   d. bone pain
   e. tremors

4. Which type of patient should not take a sodium-containing antacid?

   a. A patient with renal calculi
   b. A patient with a gastric outlet obstruction
   c. A patient with respiratory insufficiency
   d. A patient with congestive heart failure
   e. A patient with decreased kidney function

5. Which of the following drugs would have a decreased pharmacological effect when administered with an antacid?

   a. tetracycline
   b. valproic acid
   c. phenytoin
   d. ranitidine
   e. All of the above

6. Which gastrointestinal stimulant may be given IV immediately after major abdominal surgery to reduce the risk of paralytic ileus?

   a. dexpanthenol
   b. metoclopramide
   c. famotidine
   d. ranitidine
   e. cimetidine

7. Patients receiving high or prolonged doses of metoclopramide should be monitored for symptoms of ____.

   a. extrapyramidal reactions
   b. tardive dyskinesia
   c. shortness of breath
   d. Both a and b
   e. All of the above

8. Histamine H_2 antagonists ____.

   a. inhibit the action of histamine in the stomach
   b. decrease total pepsin output
   c. reduce the secretions of gastric acid
   d. Both a and c
   e. All of the above

9. Which of the following is not an example of a histamine H_2 antagonist?

   a. Reglan
   b. Zantac
   c. Tagamet
   d. Pepcid
   e. Axid

10. In which of the following patients are histamine H_2 antagonists contraindicated?

   a. A patient with diabetes
   b. A patient with renal impairment
   c. A patient with a known hypersensitivity
   d. A patient with hepatic impairment
   e. All of the above

11. With which of the following drugs, when given concurrently with a histamine H_2 antagonist, does the patient have an increased risk of toxicity?

   a. oral anticoagulant
   b. phenytoin
   c. quinidine
   d. lidocaine
   e. All of the above

12. Charcoal may be used as a(n) ____.

   a. antiflatulent
   b. antidote in poisoning
   c. method of preventing nonspecific pruritus
   d. Both a and b
   e. All of the above

13. High doses of digestive enzymes may produce ____ as an adverse effect.

   a. nausea
   b. diarrhea
   c. rash
   d. Both a and b
   e. Both b and c

14. Digestive enzymes may ____.

   a. be taken before or with meals in a capsule form
   b. be sprinkled on soft foods
   c. not be chewed if in the time-released capsule form
   d. cause nausea and diarrhea
   e. All of the above

15. A patient who has ingested a corrosive substance ____.

   a. should be given an emetic immediately
   b. should be told to eat digestive enzymes
   c. should not be given an emetic
   d. Both a and b
   e. None of the above

16. Pantoprazole and rabeprazole are examples of ____.

   a. laxatives
   b. emetics
   c. proton pump inhibitors
   d. digestive enzymes
   e. gastrointestinal stimulants

17. Chamomile has been used to ____.

   a. reduce flatulence caused by a nervous stomach
   b. treat the common cold
   c. increase appetite
   d. relieve menstrual cramps
   e. All of the above

IX. RECALL FACTS

Indicate which of the following statements are facts with an F. If the statement is not a fact, leave the line blank.

ABOUT INTERACTIONS OF MISCELLANEOUS GASTROINTESTINAL DRUGS

____ 1. Misoprostol and magnesium-containing antacids used concurrently increase the risk of diarrhea.

____ 2. Salicylate toxicity is not a risk for patients taking aspirin-containing drugs and bismuth subsalicylate concurrently.

ABOUT PATIENT MANAGEMENT ISSUES WITH DRUGS THAT AFFECT THE GASTROINTESTINAL SYSTEM

____ 1. Antacids should not be given within 2 hours before or after administration of other oral drugs.

____ 2. Oral metoclopramide should be given 30 minutes after each meal.

____ 3. Emetics are the drug of choice for all ingested poisons.

____ 4. Omeprazole should be swallowed whole before taking a meal.

X. FILL IN THE BLANKS

Fill in the blanks using words from the list below.

decreased	urinary retention	dexpanthenol	medulla	chamomile
simethicone	digestive enzymes	Robinul	diarrhea	constipation
1–2 hours	metoclopramide	pregnancy	histamine H$_2$ antagonists	duodenal ulcers
pancrelipase	pancreatin			

1. Aluminum-containing antacids may produce _____, whereas magnesium-containing antacids can produce _____.

2. Corticosteroids, digoxin, and chlorpromazine have a(n) _____ pharmacological effect when administered with an antacid.

3. _____ is an example of an anticholinergic drug used for gastrointestinal tract disorders.

4. _____ is an adverse reaction that may occur during treatment with anticholinergic drugs.

5. Oral preparations of _____ are used to treat gastric stasis.

6. A common adverse reaction to the administration of _____ is intestinal colic, which may occur within 30 minutes of administration.

7. Older adults are particularly sensitive to the effects of _____.

8. _____ works by dispersing and preventing gas pockets in the intestine.

9. _____ and _____ break down and help digest fats, starches, and proteins in food.

10. Patients who have a hypersensitivity to hog or cow proteins should not take _____.

11. Emetics are used to cause vomiting by stimulating the _____.

12. Proton pump inhibitors are an important part of the treatment of _____ caused by *Helicobacter pylori.*

13. No oral drugs should be given within _____ of an antacid.

14. Ginger is not recommended for morning sickness associated with _____.

15. _____ may produce symptoms ranging from contact dermatitis to severe anaphylactic reactions in persons hypersensitive to ragweed, asters, and chrysanthemums.

XI. LIST

List the requested number of items.

1. List five agents used to treat *Helicobacter pylori.*

    a. _____

    b. _____

    c. _____

    d. _____

    e. _____

2. List the three ways that antacids may interfere with other drugs.

    a. _____

    b. _____

    c. _____

3. List four conditions in which histamine H_2 antagonists are used for treatment.

    a. _____

    b. _____

    c. _____

    d. _____

4. List six conditions or diseases for which digestive enzymes may be prescribed.

    a. _____

    b. _____

    c. _____

    d. _____

    e. _____

    f. _____

5. List three common adverse reactions of proton pump inhibitors.

    a. _____

    b. _____

    c. _____

6. List five reasons ginger may be used.

    a. _____

    b. _____

    c. _____

    d. _____

    e. _____

XII. CLINICAL APPLICATIONS

1. Mr. K has been diagnosed with a duodenal ulcer caused by *Helicobacter pylori*. His health care provider has decided that the best option for treatment is the combination drug Helidac. Explain to Mr. K how and when to take the various drugs in the dose regimen.

XIII. CASE STUDY

Mr. S. has been prescribed pancrelipase for chronic pancreatitis. He is about to be discharged from the hospital and is being given instructions related to the drug and his condition.

1. The following are all trade names for this drug except _____.
   a. Creon
   b. Prevacid
   c. Zenpep
   d. Lipram

2. Pancrelipase is responsible for all of the following except _____.
   a. breakdown and digestion of fats in food
   b. breakdown and digestion of starches in food
   c. breakdown and digestion of proteins in food
   d. increasing the strength of the spontaneous movement of the upper gastrointestinal tract

3. Contraindications and precautions Mr. S. should be aware of with this drug include all of the following except _____.
   a. it is contraindicated in patients with hypersensitivity to hog or cow proteins
   b. calcium carbonate or magnesium hydroxide antacids may decrease the effectiveness of the enzymes
   c. digestive enzymes may decrease the absorption of oral iron preparations
   d. high doses may cause constipation

4. The following are all instructions for taking the pancrelipase except, _____.
   a. the drug should be taken after meals
   b. the drug should be taken with plenty of fluids
   c. the capsule or tablet should not be bitten or chewed
   d. if a capsule is used, it may be opened and sprinkled on a small amount of soft food that does not need to be chewed, and served at room temperature in food such as applesauce or flavored gelatin

29

Drugs That Affect the Gallbladder and Intestines

I. MATCH THE FOLLOWING

Match the generic miscellaneous gastrointestinal drug from Column A with the correct trade name from Column B.

COLUMN A

_____ 1. mesalamine

_____ 2. sulfasalazine

_____ 3. infliximab

_____ 4. olsalazine

COLUMN B

A. Azulfidine

B. Asacol

C. Dipentum

D. Remicade

II. MATCH THE FOLLOWING

Match the antidiarrheal, gallstone-solubilizing agent, or bowel evacuant drug from Column A with the correct trade name from Column B.

COLUMN A

_____ 1. difenoxin HCl with atropine

_____ 2. diphenoxylate

_____ 3. loperamide

_____ 4. chenodiol

_____ 5. polyethylene glycol

_____ 6. ursodiol

_____ 7. polyethylene glycol electrolyte solution

COLUMN B

A. Motofen

B. Imodium A-D

C. Lomotil

D. Actigall

E. MiraLax

F. CoLyte

G. Chenodiol

III. MATCH THE FOLLOWING

Match the generic laxative name from Column A with the correct trade name from Column B.

COLUMN A

_____ 1. glycerin

_____ 2. docusate calcium

_____ 3. psyllium

_____ 4. docusate sodium

_____ 5. sennosides

_____ 6. magnesium sulfate

_____ 7. lactulose

_____ 8. polycarbophil

COLUMN B

A. Colace

B. Metamucil

C. Pedia-Lax

D. Epsom salt

E. Senokot

F. Kristalose

G. FiberCon

H. Kaopectate

IV. MATCH THE FOLLOWING

Match the trade name from Column A with the correct type of drug from Column B. You may use an answer more than once.

COLUMN A

____ 1. Remicade

____ 2. Imodium A-D

____ 3. Actigall

____ 4. Dipentum

____ 5. MiraLax

____ 6. Metamucil

____ 7. Colace

____ 8. Ex-Lax

COLUMN B

A. Miscellaneous gastrointestinal drug

B. Antidiarrheal

C. Gallstone-solubilizing agent

D. Laxative

E. Bowel evacuant

V. TRUE OR FALSE

Indicate whether each statement is True (T) or False (F).

____ 1. Antidiarrheals are contraindicated in children who are younger than 2 years of age.

____ 2. Radiolucent gallstones may decrease in size when a patient is given Actigall.

____ 3. Hepatotoxicity may be an adverse reaction of prolonged use of gallstone-solubilizing drugs.

____ 4. Calcified gallstones can be safely treated with ursodiol.

____ 5. The action of all laxatives is the same.

____ 6. Mineral oil, when used as a laxative, can cause impairment of fat-soluble vitamin absorption.

VI. MULTIPLE CHOICE

Circle the letter of the best answer.

1. Loperamide is an example of a(n) ____.
   a. gastrointestinal stimulant
   b. antidiarrheal
   c. histamine H_2 antagonist
   d. antacid
   e. antiflatulent

2. The drug ____ is a narcotic-related drug that is used for the treatment of diarrhea and has a potential for drug dependency.
   a. difenoxin
   b. diphenoxylate
   c. atropine
   d. loperamide
   e. simethicone

3. Antidiarrheals are contraindicated in which of the following patients?
   a. Patients with pseudomembranous colitis
   b. Patients with abdominal pain of unknown origin
   c. Patients with obstructive jaundice
   d. Patients with *Escherichia coli*, *Salmonella*, or *Shigella* infections
   e. All of the above

4. Gallstone-solubilizing drugs may ____.
   a. suppress the production of cholesterol and cholic acid by the liver
   b. be used cautiously during pregnancy
   c. be effective for all types of gallstones
   d. rarely produce adverse reactions
   e. Both a and b

5. A patient who has had a recent myocardial infarction and should not strain during defecation may be given ____ as a laxative.
   a. mineral oil
   b. saline
   c. bulk-producing products
   d. hyperosmotic agents
   e. a fecal softener

6. A "laxative habit" can result from ____.
   a. an electrolyte imbalance
   b. prolonged use of a laxative
   c. diarrhea
   d. multiple types of laxatives being used for a short time
   e. None of the above

7. Which of the following laxatives is not a pregnancy category C drug?

    a. polycarbophil
    b. mineral oil
    c. lactulose
    d. docusate
    e. glycerin

8. Olsalazine can be used to treat ____.

    a. ulcerative colitis
    b. duodenal ulcers
    c. peptic ulcers
    d. chronic inflammatory bowel disease
    e. constipation

9. The drug ____ can be used to treat Crohn disease.

    a. infliximab
    b. olsalazine
    c. mesalamine
    d. sulfasalazine
    e. misoprostol

VII. RECALL FACTS

Indicate which of the following statements are facts with an F. If the statement is not a fact, leave the line blank.

ABOUT INTERACTIONS OF MISCELLANEOUS GASTROINTESTINAL DRUGS

____ 1. Iron absorption increases with sulfasalazine use.

____ 2. Sulfasalazine and methenamine taken concurrently increase the risk of crystalluria.

____ 3. Toxicity risk increases for patients taking sulfasalazine concurrently with oral hypoglycemic drugs.

VIII. FILL IN THE BLANKS

Fill in the blanks using words from the list below.

fat-soluble vitamins	nausea	months	diarrhea	decrease
loss of water	fluids	electrolytes	abdominal fullness	bloating
lipase	mesalamine	infliximab	ulcerative colitis	

1. Antidiarrheals _____ intestinal peristalsis.

2. Patients with chronic diarrhea are encouraged to ingest extra _____.

3. Ursodiol may require many _____ of use before results are noted.

4. Laxative use, especially high doses or prolonged use, can cause _____ and a _____ and _____.

5. Mineral oil may impair the gastrointestinal tract absorption of _____.

6. The most common adverse reactions with bowel evacuants are _____, _____, and _____.

7. Orlistat inhibits _____ in the stomach and small intestine.

8. _____ is used in the treatment of chronic inflammatory bowel disease.

9. _____ is used in Crohn disease.

10. Olsalazine is used in the treatment of _____.

IX. LIST

List the requested number of items.

1. List six types of laxatives.

   a. _____

   b. _____

   c. _____

   d. _____

   e. _____

   f. _____

2. List five symptoms of Crohn disease.

   a. _____

   b. _____

   c. _____

   d. _____

   e. _____

3. List three antidiarrheal drugs.

   a. _____

   b. _____

   c. _____

4. List five adverse reactions with chenodiol.

   a. _____

   b. _____

   c. _____

   d. _____

   e. _____

5. List four drugs that exert a topical anti-inflammatory effect in the bowel.

   a. _____

   b. _____

   c. _____

   d. _____

6. List three drugs that counteract the effectiveness of ursodiol.

   a. _____

   b. _____

   c. _____

X. CLINICAL APPLICATIONS

1. Mrs. D., age 80, has been diagnosed with gallstones. Her health care provider has decided that a gallstone-solubilizing drug is appropriate for her due to her being at poor surgical risk and having minimum symptoms. What are the key points about these drugs that Mrs. D. and her family members should know about?

XI. CASE STUDY

Mr. C., age 63, had started taking dicyclomine for his irritable bowel syndrome. The health care staff is providing him information about the medication and about irritable bowel syndrome.

1. Dicyclomine works by _____.
   a. decreasing the infiltration of inflammatory cells
   b. slowing GI motility
   c. acting on the cholinergic receptors on the smooth muscle
   d. neutralizing the biological activity of tumor necrosis factor
   e. Both b and c
   f. Both a and d

2. Adverse reactions associated with taking dicyclomine include _____.
   a. dry mouth
   b. headache
   c. constipation
   d. dizziness
   e. blurred vision
   f. Answers a, c, and d
   g. Answers a, d, and e

3. Dicyclomine is contraindicated in _____.
   a. ulcerative colitis
   b. myasthenia gravis
   c. glaucoma
   d. All of the above

4. Dicyclomine may cause dry mouth. This can be resolved by _____.
   a. sucking on hard candy
   b. ingesting more salt
   c. sucking ice chips
   d. using an artificial saliva product
   e. All of the above
   f. Answers a, c, and d

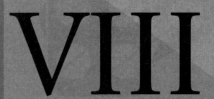

DRUGS THAT AFFECT THE ENDOCRINE AND REPRODUCTIVE SYSTEMS

VIII

30

Antidiabetic Drugs

I. MATCH THE FOLLOWING

Match the term from Column A with the correct definition from Column B.

COLUMN A

____ 1. Diabetes mellitus

____ 2. Diabetic ketoacidosis

____ 3. Glucagon

____ 4. Hyperglycemia

____ 5. Hypoglycemia

____ 6. Lipodystrophy

____ 7. Insulin

COLUMN B

A. Low blood glucose level

B. Elevated blood glucose level

C. A potentially life-threatening deficiency of insulin

D. Atrophy of subcutaneous fat

E. A hormone produced by the alpha cells of the pancreas that increases blood sugar by stimulating the conversion of glycogen to glucose in the liver

F. A chronic disorder characterized by either insufficient insulin production in the beta cells of the pancreas or by cellular resistance to insulin

G. A hormone produced by the pancreas that helps maintain blood glucose levels within normal limits

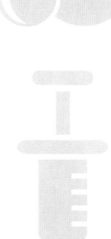

II. MATCH THE FOLLOWING

Match the generic name of insulin from Column A with the type of insulin from Column B. You may use an answer more than once.

COLUMN A

___ 1. insulin aspart protamine suspension, insulin aspart solution

___ 2. insulin lispro

___ 3. insulin injection (regular)

___ 4. insulin glargine solution

___ 5. insulin aspart solution

___ 6. insulin injection concentrate

___ 7. isophane insulin suspension and insulin inject (NPH)

___ 8. isophane insulin suspension (NPH)

COLUMN B

A. Rapid-acting

B. Intermediate-acting

C. Long-acting

D. Mixed insulin

E. High-potency insulin

F. Short-acting

III. MATCH THE FOLLOWING

Match the generic antidiabetic drug from Column A with the correct trade name from Column B.

COLUMN A

___ 1. glimepiride

___ 2. nateglinide

___ 3. miglitol

___ 4. glyburide

___ 5. pramlintide

___ 6. linagliptin

___ 7. acarbose

___ 8. sitagliptin

___ 9. metformin

___ 10. glipizide

___ 11. pioglitazone

___ 12. liraglutide

___ 13. glyburide/metformin

___ 14. rosiglitazone

COLUMN B

A. Diabeta

B. Symlin

C. Januvia

D. Starlix

E. Amaryl

F. Glyset

G. Victoza

H. Glucotrol

I. Precose

J. Glucophage

K. Tradjenta

L. Avandia

M. Glucovance

N. Actos

IV. MATCH THE FOLLOWING

Match the antidiabetic drug from Column A with the type of drug from Column B. You may use an answer more than once.

COLUMN A

____ 1. Tradjenta

____ 2. Prandin

____ 3. Amaryl

____ 4. Glyset

____ 5. Glucovance

____ 6. Byetta

____ 7. Glucophage

____ 8. Actos

____ 9. Symlin

____ 10. Precose

COLUMN B

A. Sulfonylurea

B. Alpha-glucosidase inhibitor

C. Biguanide

D. Meglitinide

E. Thiazolidinediones

F. Antidiabetic combination drug

G. Amylin analog

H. Dipeptidyl peptidase-4 inhibitor

I. Glucagon-like peptide 1 receptor agonist

V. TRUE OR FALSE

Indicate whether each statement is True (T) or False (F).

____ 1. Duetact is an antidiabetic combination drug.

____ 2. Diabetes mellitus is treated with the same drugs as diabetes insipidus.

____ 3. Type 1 diabetes is often treated with oral hypoglycemics.

____ 4. Type 2 diabetes is easier to control than type 1 diabetes.

____ 5. Human insulin is derived from a biosynthetic process using strains of *Escherichia coli*.

____ 6. Human insulin appears to cause fewer allergic reactions than insulin from animal sources.

____ 7. Hyperglycemia may occur if there is too little insulin in the bloodstream in relation to the available glucose.

____ 8. Hypoglycemic reactions are most likely to occur when insulin is at its peak activity.

____ 9. Risk factors for diabetes are gender and age.

____ 10. There is no standard dose of insulin.

____ 11. Insulin can be administered by any route.

____ 12. Lipodystrophy can interfere with the absorption of insulin from the injection site.

____ 13. Diabetic ketoacidosis results in hyperglycemia caused by a deficiency of insulin.

____ 14. Obesity is thought to contribute to type 2 diabetes by placing additional stress on the pancreas.

____ 15. Starlix is an example of a meglitinide antidiabetic drug.

____ 16. Sulfonylureas act by stimulating the beta cells of the pancreas to release insulin.

____ 17. Metformin is the only biguanide-type antidiabetic drug.

____ 18. Meglitinides act by stimulating the release of insulin from the beta cells of the pancreas.

____ 19. Starlix is an alpha-glucosidase inhibitor type of antidiabetic drug.

____ 20. Repaglinide is an example of a thiazolidinedione.

____ 21. Oral antidiabetic drugs can be used by either type 1 or type 2 diabetics with equal success.

____ 22. Adverse reactions of sulfonylureas may be reduced or eliminated by changing the dosage or giving the drug in divided doses.

____ 23. Lactic acidosis may occur with metformin use.

____ 24. The most common adverse reactions of alpha-glucosidase inhibitors are bloating and flatulence.

____ 25. Site rotation of insulin injections is crucial to prevent injury to the skin and fatty tissue.

____ 26. Meglitinides are safe to use in patients with type 1 diabetes.

____ 27. Repaglinide is safe to use during pregnancy and lactation.

____ 28. There is no fixed dosage for the treatment of diabetes.

____ 29. A patient who is stabilized with an oral antidiabetic drug but who undergoes a stressful event may require insulin.

____ 30. Acarbose and miglitol are given three times a day with the first bite of the meal.

VI. MULTIPLE CHOICE

Circle the letter of the best answer.

1. Which of the following is a glucose-elevating drug?
   a. repaglinide
   b. glucagons
   c. Glucovance
   d. glyburide
   e. Diabinese

2. Which of the following antidiabetic drugs is used as an adjunct to diet to lower blood glucose in type 2 diabetes?
   a. nateglinide
   b. NovoLog
   c. chlorpropamide
   d. Diazoxide
   e. Lantus

3. Patients with diabetes mellitus can ____.
   a. produce too much insulin
   b. produce too little insulin
   c. have cells hypersensitive to insulin
   d. have cells resistant to insulin
   e. Both b and d

4. Major adverse reactions seen with insulin administration are ____.
   a. hypoglycemia
   b. antibody development to insulin
   c. hyperglycemia
   d. allergic reactions
   e. All of the above

5. Insulin would be contraindicated in which of the following patients?
   a. A hypoglycemic patient
   b. A hyperglycemic patient
   c. A patient hypersensitive to product ingredients
   d. A lactating woman
   e. Both a and c

6. Insulin may be injected into which of the following sites?
   a. Arms
   b. Thighs
   c. Abdomen
   d. Buttocks
   e. All of the above

7. Insulin is absorbed most rapidly in the ____.
   a. upper arm
   b. abdomen
   c. thighs
   d. buttocks
   e. All sites absorb insulin equally well

8. Which of the following is not a type of oral anti-diabetic drug?
   a. Sulfonylureas
   b. Sulfonamides
   c. Biguanides
   d. Meglitinides
   e. Thiazolidinediones

9. Which of the following drugs is an example of an alpha-glucosidase inhibitor?
   a. glyburide
   b. metformin
   c. nateglinide
   d. miglitol
   e. pioglitazone

10. The drug ____ is an example of a biguanide.
    a. metformin
    a. repaglinide
    b. glimepiride
    c. acarbose
    d. rosiglitazone

11. Which of the following drugs is not a second- or third-generation sulfonylurea?
    a. glimepiride
    b. glyburide
    c. glipizide
    d. tolbutamide
    e. amaryl

12. Biguanides act by ____.
    a. stimulating the beta cells of the pancreas to produce extra insulin
    b. stimulating the beta cells of the pancreas to release insulin
    c. reducing hepatic glucose production
    d. increasing insulin sensitivity in muscle and fat cells
    e. Both c and d

13. Thiazolidinediones act by ____.
    a. increasing the release of insulin by the beta cells of the pancreas
    b. decreasing insulin resistance
    c. increasing insulin sensitivity
    d. decreasing insulin sensitivity
    e. Both b and c

14. Oral antidiabetic drugs may be ____.
    a. used in type 2 diabetics whose diet does not control their condition
    b. used with insulin in some patients
    c. used in combination (i.e., two antidiabetic drugs)
    d. Both a and c
    e. All of the above

15. Metformin ____.
    a. is sometimes given to obese diabetic patients to help with weight loss
    b. can decrease vitamin B$_{12}$ levels
    c. can cause lactic acidosis
    d. rarely causes hypoglycemia
    e. All of the above

16. Patients receiving thiazolidinediones in combination with insulin or other hypoglycemic medications are ____.
    a. at a decreased risk for hypoglycemia
    b. at an increased risk for hypoglycemia
    c. at an increased risk for hyperglycemia
    d. at a decreased risk for hyperglycemia
    e. Both a and c

17. Metformin is contraindicated in all the following patients except in ____.
    a. those who are older than 80 years of age
    b. those who are pregnant or lactating
    c. those using NSAIDs
    d. those with heart failure
    e. those with acute or chronic metabolic acidosis

18. The effects of acarbose may increase when used with all of the following drugs except with ____.
    a. digestive enzymes
    b. loop or thiazide diuretics
    c. glucocorticoids
    d. oral contraceptives
    e. calcium channel blockers

19. In which of the following conditions are alpha-glucosidase inhibitors contraindicated?
    a. Cirrhosis
    b. Hypersensitivity to the drug
    c. Diabetic ketoacidosis
    d. Chronic intestinal disease
    e. All of the above

20. All of the following drugs, when used with a meglitinide, may decrease the hypoglycemic action of the drug except ____.
    a. thiazides
    b. corticosteroids
    c. thyroid drugs
    d. salicylates
    e. sympathomimetics

21. Which of the following factors are considered when the drug regimen is determined for a diabetic?
    a. Effectiveness of the drug
    b. Tolerance of the drug
    c. Maximum recommended dosage
    d. Both a and c
    e. All of the above

22. Which of the following sulfonylureas are given 30 minutes before a meal?
    a. glipizide
    b. glyburide
    c. glimepiride
    d. tolbutamide
    e. acetohexamide

23. Secondary failure can occur when ____.
    a. there is a decreased response to a drug
    b. there is an increase in the severity of the disease
    c. sulfonylurea loses its effectiveness
    d. All of the above
    e. Both a and c

24. A patient taking an alpha-glucosidase inhibitor has a hypoglycemic reaction. Which of the following should not be given to terminate the reaction?
    a. Glucose tablets
    b. Dextrose
    c. Sugar (sucrose)
    d. Both a and b
    e. None of the above

VII. RECALL FACTS

Indicate which of the following statements are facts with an F. If the statement is not a fact, leave the line blank.

ABOUT PRODUCTS THAT MAY INCREASE THE HYPOGLYCEMIC EFFECT OF INSULIN

_____ 1. Alcohol

_____ 2. Diuretics

_____ 3. Calcium

_____ 4. Estrogen

_____ 5. Salicylates

_____ 6. Clonidine

_____ 7. Niacin

_____ 8. Tetracycline

ABOUT PRODUCTS THAT MAY DECREASE THE HYPOGLYCEMIC EFFECT OF INSULIN

_____ 1. MAOIs

_____ 2. Oral contraceptives

_____ 3. Corticosteroids

_____ 4. ACE inhibitors

_____ 5. Epinephrine

_____ 6. Beta-blocking drugs

_____ 7. Thyroid hormones

_____ 8. Albuterol

ABOUT DRUGS WITH WHICH SULFONYLUREAS WILL HAVE AN INCREASED HYPOGLYCEMIC EFFECT

_____ 1. Anticoagulants

_____ 2. Corticosteroids

_____ 3. Histamine H_2 antagonists

_____ 4. Clofibrate

_____ 5. Calcium channel blockers

_____ 6. Estrogen

_____ 7. Salicylates

_____ 8. MAOIs

VIII. FILL IN THE BLANKS

Fill in the blanks using words from the list below. You may use a word more than once.

recombinant DNA	acarbose	hypoglycemia	ketones
milk production	increase	subcutaneously	immediately
decrease	type 1 diabetes	glucometerglitazones	glucose
hypoglycemia	oral antidiabetic	initial	increased
miglitol	Glucophage XR	oral contraceptives	glimepiride
lactic acidosis	fats	coronary artery disease	

1. Insulin analogs, insulin lispro, and insulin aspart are made by using _____ technology.

2. _____ may occur when there is too much insulin in the bloodstream in relation to the available glucose.

3. Insulin appears to inhibit _____ .

4. A diabetic who is pregnant should expect her insulin requirement to _____ in the first trimester and _____ in the second and third trimester but decrease rapidly after delivery.

5. Insulin must be given by the parenteral route, usually _____ .

6. A _____ is a device used to monitor blood glucose levels.

7. Diabetic ketoacidosis results in dangerously high levels of _____ in the blood, which leads the body to begin to break down _____ , which when broken down results in _____ being produced by the liver.

8. _____ drugs are used to treat patients with type 2 diabetes but are not effective for treating _____ .

9. _____ and _____ are examples of alpha-glucosidase inhibitors.

10. Thiazolidinediones are also called _____ .

11. Biguanides can have an adverse reaction of a _____ .

12. Alpha-glucosidase inhibitors _____ the transit time of food in the digestive tract.

13. Acarbose and miglitol, when used alone, do not cause _____ .

14. First-generation sulfonylureas are contraindicated in patients with _____ or liver/kidney dysfunction.

15. There is a(n) _____ risk of lactic acidosis when metformin is used with glucocorticoids.

16. Thiazolidinediones may alter the effects of _____ .

17. Patients receiving both insulin and an oral hypoglycemic are observed often during the _____ period of therapy.

18. _____ is given once daily with the first main meal of the day.

19. _____ is given once daily with the evening meal.

20. A hypoglycemic reaction must be terminated _____ .

IX. LIST

List the requested number of items.

1. List three drugs (trade names) used as an adjunct to diet to lower blood glucose levels in type 2 diabetes.

   a. _____

   b. _____

   c. _____

2. List five risk factors for type 2 diabetes.

   a. _____

   b. _____

   c. _____

   d. _____

   e. _____

3. List three functions of insulin.

   a. _____

   b. _____

   c. _____

4. List five uses of insulin.

   a. _____

   b. _____

   c. _____

   d. _____

   e. _____

5. List five methods of ending a hypoglycemic reaction.

   a. _____

   b. _____

   c. _____

   d. _____

   e. _____

6. List six signs of hyperglycemia.

   a. _____

   b. _____

   c. _____

   d. _____

   e. _____

   f. _____

7. List eight types of antidiabetic drugs.

   a. _____

   b. _____

   c. _____

   d. _____

   e. _____

   f. _____

   g. _____

   h. _____

8. List five adverse reactions of sulfonylureas.

   a. _____

   b. _____

   c. _____

   d. _____

   e. _____

9. List the three first-generation sulfonylureas.

   a. _____

   b. _____

   c. _____

10. List five drugs that increase a patient's risk of hypoglycemia when used with metformin.

   a. _____

   b. _____

   c. _____

   d. _____

   e. _____

X. CLINICAL APPLICATIONS

1. Your neighbor suspects that her son may have type 1 diabetes. What can you tell her about this disorder?

2. You suspect that a diabetic patient who just received his or her insulin shot is having a hypoglycemic reaction. What symptoms would you expect this patient to exhibit?

XI. CASE STUDY

Mr. G. is a 43-year-old White police officer who has just been diagnosed with type 2 diabetes. He is 6'1" tall and weighs 235 lbs. His job primarily requires driving in a police car for 6 to 8 hours daily. He states that both of his parents had diabetes.

1. What risk factors does Mr. G. have for type 2 diabetes?

   a. Obesity
   b. Older age
   c. Family history of diabetes
   d. Minimal or no physical activity
   e. Race/ethnicity
   f. All of the above
   g. Answers a, c, and d

2. Mr. G.'s health care provider has put him on a diet, exercise prescription, and an oral antidiabetic medication, acarbose. When should Mr. G. take his medication?

   a. 15 minutes before meals
   b. With the first bite of the meal
   c. With or without meals
   d. Subcutaneously immediately prior to meals

3. If Mr. G. experiences hypoglycemia, what should he take?

   a. Dextrose
   b. Glucose tablet
   c. Sucrose
   d. Either a or b

31

Pituitary and Adrenocortical Hormones

I. MATCH THE FOLLOWING

Match the term from Column A with the correct definition from Column B.

COLUMN A

_____ 1. Corticosteroids

_____ 2. Diabetes insipidus

_____ 3. Glucocorticoids

_____ 4. Gonadotropins

_____ 5. Hyperstimulation syndrome

_____ 6. Somatotropic hormone

COLUMN B

A. The collective name for the glucocorticoids and mineralocorticoids

B. A disease resulting from the failure of the posterior pituitary to secrete vasopressin or from surgical removal of the pituitary

C. Sudden ovarian enlargement with accumulation of serous fluid in the peritoneal cavity

D. A hormone essential to life produced by the adrenal cortex

E. Hormones that promote growth and function of the gonads

F. A growth hormone secreted by the anterior pituitary

II. MATCH THE FOLLOWING

Match the generic drug name from Column A with the type of hormone or production site from Column B. You may use an answer more than once.

COLUMN A

_____ 1. fludrocortisone acetate

_____ 2. betamethasone

_____ 3. triamcinolone

_____ 4. desmopressin acetate

_____ 5. clomiphene citrate

_____ 6. dexamethasone

_____ 7. vasopressin

COLUMN B

A. Anterior pituitary

B. Posterior pituitary

C. Glucocorticoids

D. Mineralocorticoids

III. MATCH THE FOLLOWING

Match the generic drug name from Column A with the correct trade name from Column B.

COLUMN A

_____ 1. urofollitropin
_____ 2. prednisolone
_____ 3. corticotrophin
_____ 4. triamcinolone acetonide
_____ 5. dexamethasone
_____ 6. hydrocortisone
_____ 7. betamethasone
_____ 8. choriogonadotropin
_____ 9. vasopressin
_____ 10. clomiphene citrate

COLUMN B

A. Kenalog-10
B. Cortef
C. Acthar
D. Pitressin
E. Baycadron
F. Ovidrel
G. Celestone
H. Prelone
I. Bravelle
J. Clomid

IV. MATCH THE FOLLOWING

Match the trade name from Column A with the correct use from Column B. You may use an answer more than once.

COLUMN A

_____ 1. Clomid
_____ 2. Stimate
_____ 3. Genotropin
_____ 4. Pitressin synthetic

COLUMN B

A. Ovulatory failure
B. Growth failure
C. Diabetes insipidus

V. TRUE OR FALSE

Indicate whether each statement is True (T) or False (F).

_____ 1. Menopur and Bravelle are purified preparations extracted from the urine of postmenopausal women.

_____ 2. Multiple births and birth defects have been reported with the use of both menotropin and follitropins.

_____ 3. Urofollitropin can produce adverse reactions of hemoperitoneum and febrile reactions.

_____ 4. Menotropins are contraindicated during pregnancy.

_____ 5. There are many clinically significant interactions with the gonadotropins.

_____ 6. Gonadotropin drugs are destroyed by the gastrointestinal tract so they must be given intramuscularly or subcutaneously.

_____ 7. Somatotropic hormone may be given to children of any age regardless of epiphyseal closure.

_____ 8. Growth hormones cause few adverse reactions when administered as directed.

_____ 9. Corticotropin stimulates the anterior pituitary to produce glucocorticoids.

_____ 10. Patients taking corticotropins should avoid any vaccinations with live viruses.

_____ 11. Clomiphene therapy may be continued for up to 8 months before the drug is considered unsuccessful.

_____ 12. Desmopressin is a derivative of vasopressin.

_____ 13. Vasopressin is contraindicated in patients who have an allergy to beef or pork proteins.

____ 14. Older patients are less sensitive to the effects of vasopressin because of their decreased kidney function.

____ 15. Examples of mineralocorticoids are cortisone and prednisone.

____ 16. When a serious disease is being treated with glucocorticoids, the appearance of Cushing-like symptoms indicates that the drug should be immediately discontinued.

____ 17. Death can result from circulatory collapse if adrenal insufficiency is not treated promptly.

____ 18. Fludrocortisone acetate is the only currently available mineralocorticoid drug.

____ 19. Patients with systemic fungal infections should not receive fludrocortisone.

____ 20. A patient receiving a short-acting glucocorticoid on alternate days before 9 AM will have a greater response because of the release of additional endogenous hormone later in the day.

VI. MULTIPLE CHOICE

Circle the letter of the best answer.

1. Menotropins, when given to men, induce _____.
   a. the release of testosterone
   b. the production of sperm
   c. the inhibition of androgen release
   d. the production of prostatic secretions
   e. the male secondary sex characteristics to appear

2. The drug _____ is used to induce ovulation in women with polycystic ovarian disease.
   a. menotropin
   b. pergonal
   c. metrodin
   d. urofollitropin
   e. Both c and d

3. _____ is a synthetic, nonsteroidal compound that binds to estrogen receptors, which results in an increased secretion of follicle-stimulating hormone and luteinizing hormone.
   a. Pergonal
   b. Metrodin
   c. Clomid
   d. Protropin
   e. Humatrope

4. Clomiphene and chorionic gonadotropin are used to _____.
   a. treat prepubertal cryptorchism
   b. induce ovulation in anovulatory women
   c. treat hypogonadotropic hypogonadism
   d. treat polycystic ovaries
   e. reduce scrotal development

5. Chorionic gonadotropin administration is contraindicated in all of the following patients except in a patient with _____.
   a. liver disease
   b. precocious puberty
   c. prostatic cancer
   d. pregnancy
   e. androgen-dependent neoplasm

6. If a patient taking clomiphene complains of _____, the drug is discontinued and the health care provider is notified.
   a. ovarian stimulation or enlargement
   b. asthma
   c. migraine headaches
   d. visual disturbances
   e. Both a and d

7. In hyperstimulation syndrome, the patient may present with which of the following indicators?
   a. Anxiety
   b. Abdominal pain and distention
   c. Redness and irritation at the injection site
   d. Epilepsy
   e. Renal dysfunction

8. Corticotropin is used with caution in children because it can _____.
   a. cause scleroderma
   b. decrease the need for insulin in diabetics
   c. inhibit skeletal growth
   d. cause congestive heart failure
   e. alter kidney function

9. Vasopressin therapy may be used to _____.
   a. treat diabetes insipidus
   b. prevent and treat postoperative abdominal distention
   c. dispel gas that interferes with abdominal radiographs
   d. All of the above
   e. Both b and c

10. Pitressin Synthetic is the trade name for _____.
   a. lypressin
   b. oxytocin
   c. vasopressin
   d. desmopressin
   e. Diapid

11. The antidiuretic effect of vasopressin may be increased when taken with _____.
    a. carbamazepine
    b. alcohol
    c. heparin
    d. lithium
    e. norepinephrine

12. When being treated with vasopressin, the patient _____.
    a. may drink alcohol
    b. should measure the amount of fluids drunk each day
    c. should drink one or two glasses of water immediately after taking the drug
    d. should use the same injection site repeatedly
    e. Both b and c

13. When discontinuing glucocorticoid therapy, _____.
    a. the dosage must be tapered off over several days
    b. the dosage may be abruptly discontinued to prompt the adrenal glands to function again
    c. no tapering is required when therapy extends beyond 5 days
    d. Both b and c
    e. None of the above—glucocorticoid therapy is never discontinued

14. Adverse reactions, in addition to adrenal insufficiency, that are associated with glucocorticoid therapy may include all of the following except _____.
    a. peptic ulcers
    b. fractures
    c. infection
    d. fluid and electrolyte imbalance
    e. malabsorption syndrome

15. Glucocorticoids are contraindicated in which of the following conditions?
    a. Renal disease
    b. Serious infections
    c. Ulcerative colitis
    d. Diabetes mellitus
    e. Pregnancy

16. Fludrocortisone _____.
    a. has mineralocorticoid activity
    b. has glucocorticoid activity
    c. is used for replacement therapy for primary adrenocortical deficiency
    d. is used for replacement therapy for secondary adrenocortical deficiency
    e. All of the above

17. Mrs. P is receiving corticosteroid therapy and should be monitored regularly for which of the following?
    a. Blood pressure
    b. Signs of infection
    c. Electrolyte imbalance
    d. Mental status
    e. All of the above

18. Alternate-day administration of glucocorticoids _____.
    a. gives the patient a day of medicinal rest
    b. provides the patient with the beneficial effects of the drug while minimizing certain undesirable reactions
    c. allows the drug to be fully metabolized before the next dose
    d. keeps the anterior pituitary gland from being activated
    e. None of the above

19. Plasma levels of endogenous adrenocortical hormones are normally higher _____.
    a. between 4 PM and midnight
    b. between 8 AM and 4 PM
    c. between 2 AM and 8 AM
    d. after strenuous exercise
    e. every other day

VII. RECALL FACTS

Indicate which of the following statements are facts with an F. If the statement is not a fact, leave the line blank.

ABOUT ADVERSE REACTIONS OF CORTICOTROPINS

____ 1. Mental depression

____ 2. Hypotension

____ 3. Anorexia

____ 4. Irregular menses or amenorrhea

____ 5. Petechiae and ecchymosis

____ 6. Hirsutism

____ 7. Increased muscular strength

____ 8. Increased susceptibility to infection

____ 9. Night blindness

____ 10. Drowsiness

VIII. FILL IN THE BLANKS

Fill in the blanks using words from the list below.

infection	benzyl alcohol	urofollitropin	growth hormone
outpatient	pork	intranasal	never
glucose	water intoxication	vasopressin	menotropins
chorionic gonadotropin	adrenal insufficiency	glucocorticoids	mineralocorticoids
conserve	potassium		

1. _____ are used to induce ovulation and pregnancy in anovulatory women.

2. _____ is used to stimulate multiple follicular development in ovulatory women for in vitro fertilization.

3. The actions of _____ are identical to those of the pituitary luteinizing hormone.

4. Gonadotropins are almost always administered on a(n) _____ basis.

5. _____ is also called somatotropic hormone.

6. Protropin and humatrope are contraindicated in patients sensitive to _____.

7. Corticotropin may mask signs of _____.

8. Patients who have an allergy to _____ should not be given corticotropins.

9. _____ is secreted by the posterior pituitary gland when body fluids must be conserved.

10. _____ may be indicative of an excessive dosage of vasopressin.

11. Vasopressin and desmopressin may all be administered by the _____ route.

12. _____ is a critical deficiency of the mineralocorticoids and the glucocorticoids.

13. Mental and emotional changes may occur when _____ are administered.

14. Aldosterone and desoxycorticosterone are _____.

15. Mineralocorticoids _____ sodium and increase the excretion of _____.

16. A glucocorticoid dosage must _____ be omitted.

17. All patients receiving a glucocorticoid should have frequent checks of blood _____ levels.

IX. LIST

List the requested number of items.

1. List five patients in whom menotropins are contraindicated.

   a. _____

   b. _____

   c. _____

   d. _____

   e. _____

2. List five adverse reactions associated with clomiphene administration.

   a. _____

   b. _____

   c. _____

   d. _____

   e. _____

3. List five uses of corticotropins.

   a. _____

   b. _____

   c. _____

   d. _____

   e. _____

4. List four drugs that when taken with vasopressin can decrease its antidiuretic effect.

   a. _____

   b. _____

   c. _____

   d. _____

5. List five uses of glucocorticoids.

   a. _____

   b. _____

   c. _____

   d. _____

   e. _____

6. List five adverse reactions of mineralocorticoid therapy.

   a. _____

   b. _____

   c. _____

   d. _____

   e. _____

7. List three reasons for using caution when older patients are being treated with corticosteroids.

   a. _____

   b. _____

   c. _____

X. CLINICAL APPLICATIONS

1. Miss H. has been diagnosed with systemic lupus erythematosus (SLE) and will be receiving short-term glucocorticoid therapy as part of her initial treatment regimen. She has some concerns about how glucocorticoids will help her with this autoimmune disorder, how she should take this medication, and what sorts of adverse reactions she can expect regarding her diabetes mellitus. What can you tell her?

XI. CASE STUDY

Mr. J. is receiving desmopressin because he has recently been diagnosed with diabetes insipidus. The health care provider has prescribed an oral preparation for him.

1. Adverse reactions to vasopressin that Mr. J. should report include _____.

   a. tremor

   b. sweating

   c. vertigo

   d. All of the above

2. The adverse reactions to vasopressin that may be decreased by taking the drug after drinking one or two glasses of water include which of the following?

   a. Skin blanching

   b. Abdominal cramps

   c. Nausea

   d. Headaches

   e. Both a and d

   f. Answers a, b, and c

3. Which of the following key points about vasopressin that Mr. J. and his family need to be aware of?

   a. Drink one or two glasses of water immediately before taking the drug

   b. Measure the amount of fluids drank each day

   c. Measure the amount of urine passed at each voiding and then the amount for each 24 hour period

   d. All of the above

   e. None of the above

32

Thyroid and Antithyroid Drugs

I. MATCH THE FOLLOWING

Match the term from Column A with the correct definition from Column B.

COLUMN A

____ 1. Euthyroid
____ 2. Myxedema
____ 3. Thyroid storm
____ 4. Thyrotoxicosis
____ 5. Triiodothyronine
____ 6. Thyroxine
____ 7. Iodism
____ 8. Hypothyroidism
____ 9. Hyperthyroidism
____ 10. Goiter

COLUMN B

A. An increase in the amount of thyroid hormones secreted
B. A normal thyroid
C. A severe hypothyroidism manifested by a variety of symptoms
D. A severe form of hyperthyroidism also known as thyroid storm
E. A hormone manufactured and secreted by the thyroid gland
F. A severe form of hyperthyroidism also known as thyrotoxicosis
G. Enlargement of the thyroid gland
H. A decrease in the amount of thyroid hormone secreted
I. Excessive amounts of iodine in the body
J. A hormone manufactured and secreted by the thyroid gland

II. MATCH THE FOLLOWING

Match the generic drug name from Column A with the correct trade name from Column B.

COLUMN A

____ 1. levothyroxine sodium
____ 2. liothyronine
____ 3. liotrix
____ 4. thyroid desiccated
____ 5. methimazole
____ 6. radioactive iodine
____ 7. potassium iodide

COLUMN B

A. Tapazole
B. Thyrolar
C. Levothroid
D. Cytomel
E. Lugol Solution
F. Hicon
G. Armour Thyroid

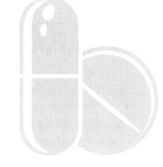

III. MATCH THE FOLLOWING

Match the trade name from Column A with the correct use from Column B. You may use an answer more than once.

COLUMN A

____ 1. Levothyroid

____ 2. Tapazole

____ 3. Hicon

____ 4. Liothyronine sodium

____ 5. Liotrix

____ 6. Iosat

____ 7. Armour

COLUMN B

A. Hypothyroidism

B. Hyperthyroidism

IV. TRUE OR FALSE

Indicate whether each statement is True (T) or False (F).

____ 1. The most common adverse reactions of thyroid hormone therapy are signs of overdose and hyperthyroidism.

____ 2. Older adults are more likely to experience adverse reactions to thyroid replacement therapy.

____ 3. Radioactive iodine is used to treat hypothyroidism.

____ 4. Generally speaking, synthetic thyroid hormones are preferred medically because they are more uniform in potency than natural hormones.

____ 5. Levothyroxine is the drug of choice for hypothyroidism.

____ 6. For best results, thyroid hormones should be administered once-a-day, early in the morning, and on an empty stomach.

____ 7. Thyroid replacement therapy is for life.

____ 8. The therapeutic effects of antithyroid drugs are seen immediately since they neutralize existing thyroid hormones in circulation and storage.

____ 9. An oral solution of Lugol's may be given to a patient to help prepare him or her for thyroid surgery.

____ 10. Iodine solutions should be drunk through a straw to avoid tooth discoloration.

V. MULTIPLE CHOICE

Circle the letter of the best answer.

1. Synthetic hormones are the drugs of choice for hypothyroidism for all of the following reasons except that they ____.
   a. are difficult for the patient to manage
   b. require once-a-day dosing
   c. have a more uniform potency than other drugs
   d. are a synthetic form of the hormone

2. Which of the following are signs of hyperthyroidism?
   a. Flushed, warm, moist skin
   b. Moderate hypertension
   c. Tachycardia
   d. Elevated body temperature
   e. All of the Above

3. In which of the following patients are thyroid hormones contraindicated?
   a. Pregnant women
   b. Lactating women
   c. After recent myocardial infarction
   d. Patients with Addison disease
   e. Elderly men

4. A patient receiving thyroid hormones may experience a decreased effectiveness of ____.
   a. digitalis
   b. oral anticoagulants
   c. oral contraceptives
   d. antacids
   e. live vaccines

5. Drugs used for the medical management of hyper-thyroidism include ____.
   a. propylthiouracil
   b. Tapazole
   c. PTU
   d. methimazole
   e. All of the Above

6. Patients taking antithyroid drugs should be moni-tored for ____.
   a. signs of infection
   b. hypercoagulation
   c. liver dysfunction
   d. visual disturbances
   e. ototoxicity

7. When iodine solutions are administered, the patient should be closely monitored for symptoms of ____.
   a. iodism
   b. swelling around the mouth
   c. difficulty breathing
   d. iodine allergy
   e. All of the above

8. Radioactive iodine ____.
   a. is given orally as a single dose
   b. effects occur within 24 hours
   c. requires the patient to remain inactive
   d. frequently causes a thyroid storm to occur
   e. Both a and b

VI. RECALL FACTS

Indicate which of the following statements are facts with an F. If the statement is not a fact, leave the line blank.

ABOUT USES OF ANTITHYROID DRUGS

____ 1. Hyperthyroidism

____ 2. Carcinoma of the Thyroid

____ 3. Graves disease

____ 4. Pituitary thyroid-stimulating hormone suppression

____ 5. Preparation for thyroid surgery for hyperthy-roid patients

____ 6. Thyrotoxic crisis

VII. FILL IN THE BLANKS

Fill in the blanks using words from the list below

contraindicated   agranulocytosis   A   additive   iodism   hyperthyroidism

1. Thyroid hormones are classified as Pregnancy Category _____ drugs and are considered safe to use during pregnancy.

2. Antithyroid drugs or thyroid antagonists are used to treat _____.

3. _____ is the most serious adverse reaction associated with methimazole and propylthiouracil.

4. Adverse reactions that occur with the use of strong iodine solutions can include symptoms of _____.

5. Radioactive iodine is _____ during pregnancy and lactation.

6. When methimazole and propylthiouracil are administered with other bone marrow depres-sants, there can be a(n) _____ effect on the bone marrow.

VIII. LIST

List the requested number of items.

1. List four uses of thyroid hormones.

   a. _____

   b. _____

   c. _____

   d. _____

2. List five adverse reactions seen after the administration of radioactive iodine.

   a. _____

   b. _____

   c. _____

   d. _____

   e. _____

3. List four antithyroid preparations.

   a. _____

   b. _____

   c. _____

   d. _____

4. List five symptoms of myxedema.

   a. _____

   b. _____

   c. _____

   d. _____

   e. _____

IX. CLINICAL APPLICATIONS

1. Mrs. T, age 47, has been diagnosed with Hashimoto thyroiditis and will soon begin thyroid hormone treatment for this hypothyroid condition. Her health care provider has prescribed Synthroid and wants you to go over the signs of hyperthyroidism with Mrs. T. Explain to Mrs. T why she should be concerned about hyperthyroidism when she has hypothyroidism.

X. CASE STUDY

Mr. G., age 61, is now taking Tapazole for management of his hyperthyroidism. Tapazole inhibits the manufacture of thyroid hormones. Mr. G. is wondering about how the medication will work and what he can expect.

1. Tapazole _____.
   a. does not affect existing thyroid hormones that are circulating in the blood
   b. effects may not be observed for 3 to 4 weeks
   c. Both a and b are true
   d. Both a and b are false

2. Which of the following is true about Tapazole?
   a. The drug should be taken at regular intervals around the clock.
   b. The drug should not be taken in larger doses or more frequently than directed.
   c. The patient should record his weight twice per week and notify the health care provider if there is a sudden weight gain or loss.
   d. All of the Above.
   e. None of the Above.

3. Adverse effects of Tapazole include _____.
   a. agranulocytosis
   b. loss of hair
   c. arthralgia
   d. tachycardia
   e. All of the above
   f. Answers a, b, and c

33

Male and Female Hormones and Drugs for Erectile Dysfunction

I. MATCH THE FOLLOWING

Match the term from Column A with the correct definition from Column B.

COLUMN A

_____ 1. Androgens

_____ 2. Estradiol

_____ 3. Estrogens

_____ 4. Priapism

_____ 5. Progesterone

_____ 6. Progestins

_____ 7. Testosterone

_____ 8. Virilization

COLUMN B

A. Acquisition of male sexual characteristics by a woman

B. Female hormones influenced by the anterior pituitary gland

C. Prolonged erection accompanied by pain and tenderness

D. The most potent of the three endogenous estrogens

E. Hormones that stimulate activity of the accessory male sex organs

F. The most potent naturally occurring androgen

G. Female hormones influenced by the anterior pituitary gland

H. Natural or synthetic substances that cause changes similar to those of progesterones

II. MATCH THE FOLLOWING

Match the generic drug name from Column A with the type of hormone or production site from Column B. You may use an answer more than once.

COLUMN A

___ 1. conjugated estrogen

___ 2. danazol

___ 3. testosterone buccal

___ 4. estradiol

___ 5. hydroxyprogesterone caproate

___ 6. norethindrone

___ 7. estropipate

___ 8. fluoxymesterone

___ 9. progesterone

___ 10. megestrol acetate

___ 11. methyltestosterone

___ 12. medroxyprogesterone acetate

COLUMN B

A. Androgens

B. Estrogens

C. Progestins

III. MATCH THE FOLLOWING

Match the generic drug name from Column A with the correct trade name from Column B.

COLUMN A

___ 1. fluoxymesterone

___ 2. methyltestosterone

___ 3. testosterone buccal

___ 4. testosterone enanthate

___ 5. conjugated estrogens

___ 6. esterified estrogens

___ 7. estradiol oral

___ 8. estradiol transdermal patch

___ 9. estradiol vaginal tablet

___ 10. estropipate

___ 11. hydroxyprogesterone caproate

___ 12. megestrol acetate

___ 13. norethindrone

___ 14. progesterone oral

COLUMN B

A. Striant

B. Premarin

C. Estrace

D. Prometrium

E. Aygestin

F. Androxy

G. Vagifem

H. Ogen

I. Makena

J. Android

K. Menest

L. Megace ES

M. Alora

N. Delastryl

IV. MATCH THE FOLLOWING

Match the trade name from Column A with the correct use from Column B. You may use an answer more than once.

COLUMN A

_____ 1. Android

_____ 2. Estratest

_____ 3. Premarin

_____ 4. Prometrium

_____ 5. Enjuvia

_____ 6. Testopel

_____ 7. Delastryl

_____ 8. Striant

_____ 9. Megace

_____ 10. Menest

_____ 11. Crinone

_____ 12. Aygestin

COLUMN B

A. Inoperable breast cancer

B. Vasomotor symptoms

C. Amenorrhea

D. Male hypogonadism

V. MATCH THE FOLLOWING

Match the trade name of the drug from Column A with the type of drug from Column B. You may use an answer more than once.

COLUMN A

_____ 1. Anadrol-50

_____ 2. Propecia

_____ 3. Avodart

_____ 4. Oxandrin

COLUMN B

A. Anabolic steroids

B. Androgen hormone inhibitors

VI. TRUE OR FALSE

Indicate whether each statement is True (T) or False (F).

_____ 1. Virilization is one of the most common adverse reactions in women receiving an androgen preparation for breast cancer.

_____ 2. Illegal use of anabolic steroids in young, healthy individuals has resulted in deaths.

_____ 3. Prolonged high-dose anabolic steroid use can become psychologically and possibly physically addicting.

_____ 4. Older men treated with anabolic steroids are at no higher risk for prostatic enlargement and prostate cancer than younger men.

_____ 5. Proscar use results in a decrease in the size of the prostate gland and therefore is used to treat the symptoms of benign prostatic hypertrophy.

_____ 6. Adverse reactions to finasteride are usually mild and do not require discontinuation of the drug.

_____ 7. Anabolic steroid or androgen use by older adults with cardiac problems or kidney disease results in an increased risk for sodium and water retention.

_____ 8. Synthetic progestins are preferred for medical use.

_____ 9. Estrogens have few adverse reactions when given by the correct route.

_____ 10. Cigarette smoking increases the risk for cardiovascular complications in patients receiving estrogen therapy.

_____ 11. Oral estrogens are administered with food or immediately after eating to reduce gastrointestinal upset.

_____ 12. Medroxyprogesterone acetate is used in the treatment of abnormal uterine bleeding, secondary amenorrhea, and as a contraceptive.

_____ 13. Black cohosh is thought to increase diminished estrogen levels in menopausal women.

_____ 14. Saw palmetto is used to treat benign prostatic hypertrophy.

VII. MULTIPLE CHOICE

Circle the letter of the best answer.

1. Androgen therapy in males is used for ____.
   a. treatment of hypergonadism
   b. replacement therapy for testosterone deficiency
   c. treatment of precocious puberty
   d. inhibition of testicular development
   e. as part of a treatment regimen in men who have prostatic tumors

2. Adverse reactions of males to androgen therapy may include which of the following?
   a. Fluid and electrolyte imbalances
   b. Virilization
   c. Hair regrowth
   d. Clearing of acne
   e. Testicular enlargement

3. Anabolic steroids work by ____.
   a. decreasing endogenous production of androgens
   b. imitating the action of glucocorticoids
   c. stimulating androgen release
   d. promoting tissue building processes
   e. blocking the action of estrogen

4. Proscar ____.
   a. is a synthetic compound drug
   b. is an androgen hormone inhibitor
   c. has a generic name of finasteride
   d. inhibits the conversion of testosterone into 5 alpha-dihydrotestosterone
   e. All of the Above

5. An example of a progestin is ____.
   a. Ortho-Est
   b. Aygestin
   c. Estrace
   d. Proscar
   e. Oreton Methyl

6. Which of the following is not an endogenous estrogen?
   a. estradiol
   b. estriol
   c. estrone
   d. progesterone
   e. both a and b

7. All of the following are uses for progestins except:
   a. Inoperable breast cancer
   b. Treatment of amenorrhea
   c. Treatment of endometriosis
   d. Treatment of functional uterine bleeding
   e. Oral contraceptives

8. Warnings associated with the use of estrogens include increased risk of ____.
   a. endometrial cancer
   b. gallbladder disease
   c. hypertension
   d. thromboembolic disease
   e. All of the above

9. In which of the following conditions are progestins contraindicated?
   a. Thromboembolic disorders
   b. Pregnancy
   c. Cerebral hemorrhage
   d. Impaired liver function
   e. All of the Above

10. Combination oral contraceptives have ____ warnings associated with their use as do estrogens and progestins.
    a. increased
    b. the same
    c. decreased
    d. All of the Above
    e. None of the Above

11. Mrs. R forgot to take her oral contraceptive on Tuesday. She then took two doses on Wednesday to make up for the missed dose. Because of this Mrs. R ____.
    a. has no increased chance of pregnancy
    b. has an increased chance of pregnancy
    c. should discontinue the oral contraceptives for the rest of the month
    d. may require a higher dose to be prescribed next month
    e. Answers b and d

12. Black cohosh ____.
    a. has a primary adverse effect of nausea
    b. should not be taken by pregnant women
    c. may reduce physical and psychological symptoms associated with menopause
    d. All of the Above

13. The most common adverse reaction of phosphodiesterase type 5 inhibitors is ____.
    a. headache
    b. nausea
    c. impairment of color discrimination
    d. bleeding
    e. Both a and c

14. Emergency contraception _____.
   a. is used when unprotected intercourse occurs to prevent pregnancy
   b. contains a progestin
   c. prevents ovulation
   d. All of the Above

15. All of the following are names of emergency contraceptives except _____.
   a. Next Choice
   b. Makena
   c. Plan B
   d. Plan B One-Step
   e. Ella

VIII. RECALL FACTS

Indicate which of the following statements are facts with an F. If the statement is not a fact, leave the line blank.

ABOUT USES OF ESTROGEN

____ 1. Used in combination with progesterones as contraceptives
____ 2. Used in combination with progesterones in hormone replacement therapy in postmenopausal women
____ 3. Female hypergonadism
____ 4. Relieve vasomotor symptoms of menopause
____ 5. Selected cases of inoperable breast carcinoma
____ 6. Palliative treatment for advanced prostatic carcinoma
____ 7. Atrophic vaginitis
____ 8. Osteoporosis in women past menopause

ABOUT ADVERSE REACTIONS OF PROGESTINS

____ 1. Amenorrhea
____ 2. Breakthrough bleeding
____ 3. Melasma
____ 4. Mental stimulation
____ 5. Decrease in acne
____ 6. Edema
____ 7. Spotting
____ 8. Breast enlargement

IX. FILL IN THE BLANKS

Fill in the blanks using words from the list below.

X	slow	Implanon	finasterideestradiol	decreased
3	saw palmetto	virilization	balancethromboembolic	prostaglandins
counteracts	rapid	phosphodiesterase type 5		

1. Androgen therapy for women with hormone-dependent malignant breast tumors _____ the effect of estrogen on these tumors.

2. _____ is the most common adverse reaction in women associated with anabolic steroid use.

3. Anabolic steroids are classified as a Pregnancy Category _____ drug.

4. _____ can be used to help prevent male pattern baldness in men with early signs of hair loss.

5. _____ is the most potent estrogen.

6. Adverse reactions of estrogen/progestin combinations as oral contraceptives can be minimized by adjusting the estrogen/progestin _____.

7. Oral contraceptives should be discontinued at least 4 weeks before a surgical procedure or prolonged immobilization to avoid _____ complications.

8. The effects of the progestins are _____ when administered with an anticonvulsant, barbiturate, or rifampin.

9. With prostatic carcinoma, the response to female hormone therapy may be _____, but with breast carcinoma, the response is usually _____.

10. The contraceptive implant Etonogestrel is also called _____.

11. Depo-Provera is given intramuscularly every _____ months.

12. _____, an herb, is used to treat benign prostatic hypertrophy.

13. Two types of drugs used to treat erectile dysfunction are the _____ inhibitors and the _____.

X. LIST

List the requested number of items.

1. List four intended uses of anabolic steroids

    a. _____

    b. _____

    c. _____

    d. _____

2. List five actions of estrogens.

    a. _____

    b. _____

    c. _____

    d. _____

    e. _____

3. List the four types of estrogen and progestin oral contraceptives.

    a. _____

    b. _____

    c. _____

    d. _____

4. List four common adverse reactions of female hormones.

    a. _____

    b. _____

    c. _____

    d. _____

5. List five conditions, other than known hypersensitivity, in which estrogen therapy is contraindicated.

    a. _____

    b. _____

    c. _____

    d. _____

    e. _____

XI. CLINICAL APPLICATIONS

1. Mr. J is taking a phosphodiesterase 5 inhibitor for erectile dysfunction. He wants to know more about these drugs. What are some important facts he needs to be aware of when he is taking a phosphodiesterase 5 inhibitor?

XII. CASE STUDY

Ms. L. is taking an estrogen medication for relief of the vasomotor symptoms of menopause and for osteoporosis prevention. She is being given information about the medication before she is sent home.

1. Which of the following is true if she experiences gastrointestinal upset while taking the drug?

    a. She should take the drug on an empty stomach.
    b. She should take the drug with food.
    c. She should take the drug two hours after eating.
    d. None of Above.

2. Ms. L. should notify her health care provider if she experiences ____.

    a. pain in the legs or groin area
    b. sharp chest pain or sudden shortness of breath
    c. lumps in the breast
    d. sudden severe headache
    e. Any of the above

3. Ms. L. has diabetes. What should she be told about the use of estrogens and diabetes?

    a. She should check her blood glucose daily or more often.
    b. She should contact her health care provider if her blood glucose is elevated.
    c. She may ignore elevated blood glucose for up to three days and see if she has an adverse reaction.
    d. Both a and b.

34

Uterine Drugs

I. MATCH THE FOLLOWING

Match the term from Column A with the correct definition from Column B.

COLUMN A

___ 1. Uterine atony

___ 2. Ergotism

___ 3. Oxytocic drugs

___ 4. Oxytocin

COLUMN B

A. An overdose of ergonovine

B. Used before birth to induce uterine contractions similar to those of normal labor

C. An endogenous hormone produced by the posterior pituitary gland

D. Marked relaxation of the uterine muscle

II. MATCH THE FOLLOWING

Match the generic drug from Column A with the correct trade name from Column B.

COLUMN A

___ 1. methylergonovine

___ 2. oxytocin

___ 3. carboprost

___ 4. dinoprostone

___ 5. mifepristone

COLUMN B

A. Hemabate

B. Cervidil

C. Mifeprex

D. Pitocin

E. Methergine

III. MATCH THE FOLLOWING

Match the drug from Column A with the correct use from Column B. You may use an answer more than once.

COLUMN A

___ 1. Mifeprex

___ 2. Methergine

___ 3. Pitocin

___ 4. Cervidil

___ 5. Hemabate

COLUMN B

A. Termination of an intrauterine pregnancy

B. Uterine atony and hemorrhage

C. Antepartum to initiate or improve uterine contractions

IV. MATCH THE FOLLOWING

Match the use of oxytocin from Column A to its route of administration from Column B. You may use an answer more than once.

COLUMN A

____ 1. Stimulate milk ejection

____ 2. Control postpartum bleeding

____ 3. Starting labor

____ 4. Produce uterine contractions in the third stage of labor

____ 5. Management of incomplete abortion

COLUMN B

A. IV

B. IM

C. Intranasally

V. TRUE OR FALSE

Indicate whether each statement is True (T) or False (F).

____ 1. An oxytocic drug is used to stimulate the uterus.

____ 2. Methylergonovine works by decreasing the strength, duration, and frequency of contractions.

____ 3. Methylergonovine is used to prevent postpartum and postabortal hemorrhage caused by uterine atony.

____ 4. Abdominal cramping after ergonovine administration indicates that the drug is effective.

____ 5. Methylergonovine can be used to induce labor.

____ 6. Ergonovine may be administered IV or IM.

____ 7. The exact mechanism of action of oxytocin in normal labor is clearly understood.

____ 8. It is imperative to discontinue the administration of oxytocin when any adverse reactions are reported.

____ 9. Excessive stimulation of the uterus can result in uterine rupture or uterine hypertonicity.

VI. MULTIPLE CHOICE

Circle the letter of the best answer.

1. Ergonovine ____.
   a. increases the strength of uterine contractions
   b. increases the frequency of uterine contractions
   c. increases the duration of uterine contractions
   d. decreases uterine bleeding
   e. All of the Above

2. A patient who is calcium deficient and receiving ergonovine may ____.
   a. not respond to the drug
   b. respond to the drug if given IV calcium
   c. over respond to the drug
   d. go into calcium shock
   e. Both a and b

3. In which instance(s) is ergonovine contraindicated?
   a. Known hypersensitivity
   b. Hypertension
   c. Before delivery of the placenta
   d. Both a and b
   e. All of the Above

4. Methylergonovine is contraindicated in all of the following patients except ____.
   a. hypertension
   b. preeclampsia
   c. known hypersensitivity
   d. All of the Above
   e. Both a and c

5. Methylergonovine is usually ____.
   a. given IM
   b. given after the delivery of the placenta
   c. given at the time the anterior shoulder is delivered
   d. All of the above
   e. Both a and c

6. Oxytocin may be administered by the ____ route.
   a. intravenous
   b. intranasal
   c. intramuscular
   d. All of the Above
   e. None of the Above; it is given only by the oral route.

VII. RECALL FACTS

Indicate which of the following statements are facts with an F. If the statement is not a fact, leave the line blank.

ABOUT ADVERSE REACTIONS ASSOCIATED WITH ERGONOVINE AND METHYLERGONOVINE

____ 1. Bradycardia

____ 2. Numb fingers or toes

____ 3. Dizziness

____ 4. Water intoxication

____ 5. Double vision

____ 6. Nausea and vomiting

____ 7. Anorexia

____ 8. Elevated blood pressure

____ 9. Temporary chest pain

____ 10. Red, swollen tongue

ABOUT CONDITIONS IN WHICH OXYTOCIN IS CONTRAINDICATED

____ 1. Hypersensitivity

____ 2. Cephalopelvic disproportion

____ 3. Total placenta previa

____ 4. Hypertension

____ 5. Severe toxemia

____ 6. Hypertonic uterus

____ 7. Digitalis toxicity

____ 8. Obstetric emergencies

VIII. FILL IN THE BLANKS

Fill in the blanks using words from the list below.

intravenous	short	discontinued	ergotism
before	after	water intoxication	calcium deficient

1. Oxytocic drugs are used _____ birth.

2. Ergonovine is given _____ the delivery of the placenta.

3. _____ is an overdosage of ergonovine which in severe cases can result in coma.

4. Patients who are _____ may not respond to ergonovine.

5. When ergotism occurs, ergonovine must be _____.

6. Methylergonovine is not usually given by the _____ route as it can cause stroke or sudden hypertension.

7. Oxytocin is a _____ acting drug.

8. Intravenous oxytocin can cause _____ because of the antidiuretic effect of the drug.

IX. LIST

List the requested number of items.

1. List the three uses of uterine drugs.

    a. _____

    b. _____

    c. _____

2. List the three drugs that can be used to stimulate the uterus.

    a. _____

    b. _____

    c. _____

3. List four symptoms of ergotism.

a. _____

b. _____

c. _____

d. _____

4. List the three effects of oxytocin.

a. _____

b. _____

c. _____

5. List five adverse reactions of oxytocin.

a. _____

b. _____

c. _____

d. _____

e. _____

X. CLINICAL APPLICATIONS

1. Ms. P has been given ergonovine for postpartum hemorrhage. As a health care worker involved in her case, you note that her heart rate has reached 120 beats/minute, and she is complaining of tingling of the extremities and chest pain. What should you do in response to this information? What trouble might Ms. P be having?

XI. CASE STUDY

Ms. J. is in labor and receiving oxytocin intravenously. She is complaining that her contractions are occurring with much more force than earlier, though not more frequently, and she is very uncomfortable.

1. Ms. J. could be experiencing ____.
   a. hyperstimulation of the uterus
   b. water intoxication
   c. ergotism
   d. hypertension

2. Hyperstimulation of the uterus during labor may lead to ____.
   a. uterine tetany
   b. marked impairment of uteroplacental blood flow
   c. uterine rupture
   d. cervical rupture

   e. amniotic fluid embolism
   f. trauma to the infant
   g. All of the Above

3. Overstimulation of the uterus is dangerous to both the fetus and the mother and can occur ____.
   a. in a uterus that is hypersensitive to oxytocin
   b. even when the drug is administered properly
   c. when metabolism by cytochrome P4503A4 is occurring
   d. All of the above
   e. Both a and b

ANTI-INFECTIVE DRUGS

IX

35

Antibacterial Drugs

I. MATCH THE FOLLOWING

Match the term from Column A with the correct definition from Column B.

COLUMN A

___ 1. Anaphylactoid reaction

___ 2. Antibacterial

___ 3. Anti-infective

___ 4. Bactericidal

___ 5. Bacteriostatic

___ 6. Cross-allergenicity

___ 7. Cross-sensitivity

___ 8. Penicillinase

___ 9. Prophylaxis

___ 10. Stevens-Johnson syndrome

___ 11. Superinfection

COLUMN B

A. Active against bacteria

B. Another word for antibacterial; drugs used to treat infections and bacteria

C. Serious allergic reaction to a drug, which initially exhibits reactions easily confused with less severe disorders

D. Synonymous with cross-allergenicity

E. An enzyme that inactivates penicillin

F. Unusual or exaggerated allergic reaction

G. An agent or drug that destroys bacteria

H. An overgrowth of bacterial or fungal microorganisms not affected by the antibiotic being used for treatment

I. Allergy to drugs in the same or related group

J. Prevention

K. Drugs that slow or retard the multiplication of bacteria

II. MATCH THE FOLLOWING

Match the generic name of sulfonamide, penicillin, or cephalosporin from Column A with the correct trade name from Column B.

COLUMN A

___ 1. mafenide
___ 2. penicillin G (aqueous)
___ 3. trimethoprim and sulfamethoxazole
___ 4. cefotaxime
___ 5. amoxicillin and clavulanate potassium
___ 6. oxacillin
___ 7. cefdinir
___ 8. cefixime
___ 9. amoxicillin
___ 10. silver sulfadiazine
___ 11. cefpodoxime
___ 12. ticarcillin/clavulanate
___ 13. ceftriaxone
___ 14. ampicillin/sulbactam
___ 15. cephalexin

COLUMN B

A. Bactrim
B. Claforan
C. Timentin
D. Unasyn
E. Omnicef
F. Sulfamylon
G. Bactocill
H. Rocephin
I. Silvadene
J. Maxataq
K. Keflex
L. Pfizerpen
M. Vantin
N. Suprax
O. Augmentin

III. MATCH THE FOLLOWING

Match the generic name of tetracycline, macrolide, or lincosamide from Column A with the correct trade name from Column B.

COLUMN A

___ 1. demeclocycline
___ 2. clindamycin
___ 3. clarithromycin
___ 4. azithromycin
___ 5. minocycline
___ 6. doxycycline
___ 7. lincomycin
___ 8. erythromycin ethylsuccinate

COLUMN B

A. Biaxin
B. Cleocin
C. Minocin
D. EryPed
E. Vibramycin
F. Zithromax
G. Lincocin
H. Declomycin

IV. MATCH THE FOLLOWING

Match the generic name of fluoroquinolone or aminoglycoside from Column A with the correct trade name from Column B.

COLUMN A

____ 1. gemifloxacin

____ 2. ofloxacin

____ 3. ciprofloxacin

____ 4. norfloxacin

____ 5. moxifloxacin

____ 6. gentamicin

____ 7. levofloxacin

____ 8. tobramycin

COLUMN B

A. Levaquin

B. Factive

C. Noroxin

D. Tobrex

E. Avelox

F. Garamycin

G. Floxin

H. Cipro

V. MATCH THE FOLLOWING

Match the trade name of the drug from Column A to the drug category from Column B. You may use an answer more than once.

COLUMN A

____ 1. Timentin

____ 2. Lincocin

____ 3. Keflex

____ 4. sulfadiazine

____ 5. Vibramycin

____ 6. Augmentin

____ 7. Claforan

____ 8. Bicillin

____ 9. Suprax

____ 10. Bactocill

____ 11. Zithromax

____ 12. Silvadene

____ 13. Tobrex

____ 14. Cipro

____ 15. Fortez

____ 16. Bactrim

____ 17. Ceftin

____ 18. Omnicef

____ 19. Spectracef

____ 20. Zosyn

____ 21. Maxipime

____ 22. Teflaro

____ 23. Biaxin

COLUMN B

A. Sulfonamide—single agent

B. Sulfonamide—multiple preparation

C. Miscellaneous sulfonamide preparation

D. Natural penicillin

E. Penicillinase-resistant penicillins

F. Aminopenicillin

G. Extended-spectrum penicillin

H. First-generation cephalosporin

I. Second-generation cephalosporin

J. Third-generation cephalosporin

K. Fourth-generation cephalosporin

L. Fifth-generation cephalosporin

M. Tetracycline

N. Macrolide

O. Lincosamide

P. Fluoroquinolone

Q. Aminoglycoside

VI. TRUE OR FALSE

Indicate whether each statement is True (T) or False (F).

____ 1. Penicillins were the first antibiotic drug developed that effectively treated infections.

____ 2. Crystalluria associated with sulfonamide use may be prevented by increasing fluid intake during therapy.

____ 3. Stevens-Johnson syndrome can be fatal.

____ 4. Sulfonamides are a Pregnancy Category C drug and therefore are safe to use during any stage of pregnancy.

____ 5. A patient taking a sulfonamide drug almost always has an active infection.

____ 6. Older adults generally have fewer complications with sulfonamides than do younger adults.

____ 7. Natural penicillins are less effective than some of the newer antibiotics for treating a broad range of infections.

____ 8. Beta-lactamase inhibitors are as effective alone as antibiotics.

____ 9. Penicillins act by preventing bacteria from using a substance that is necessary for the maintenance of the bacteria's outer cell wall.

____ 10. Penicillins may be bacteriostatic or bactericidal.

____ 11. Penicillins are the only antibiotics effective in treating viral and fungal infections.

____ 12. Glossitis and stomatitis are adverse reactions sometimes seen with oral penicillin administration.

____ 13. Patients with an allergy to one penicillin are most likely allergic to all penicillins and have a higher incidence of allergy to the cephalosporins.

____ 14. Superinfections may occur with the use of any antibiotic and are potentially life threatening.

____ 15. Symptoms of candidiasis can include lesions in the mouth or anal/genital itching.

____ 16. A black, furry tongue may be a sign of a fungal superinfection caused by oral penicillin use.

____ 17. Penicillin absorption is not affected by food, so it may be taken without regard to meals.

____ 18. Cephalosporins are bacteriostatic.

____ 19. Cephalosporins may be given prophylactically to patients undergoing gastrointestinal or vaginal surgery.

____ 20. Therapy with cephalosporins may result in bacterial or fungal superinfections.

____ 21. Frequent liquid stools in patients receiving cephalosporin therapy indicate that the medication is effectively working.

____ 22. Tetracyclines, macrolides, and lincosamides are considered to be broad-spectrum antibiotics.

____ 23. Tetracyclines are bactericidal.

____ 24. Tetracyclines work by inhibiting bacterial protein synthesis.

____ 25. Tetracyclines may cause a photosensitivity reaction.

____ 26. Tetracyclines are safe to give during pregnancy.

____ 27. Macrolides are particularly effective in treating infections of the respiratory and genital tracts.

____ 28. Macrolides are safe to use as prophylaxis in patients allergic to penicillins.

____ 29. All of the macrolides cause severe gastrointestinal disturbances.

____ 30. Macrolides may cause pseudomembranous colitis.

____ 31. Lincosamides act by inhibiting protein synthesis.

____ 32. Lincosamides are effective against gram-positive and gram-negative microorganisms.

____ 33. Lincosamides have a high potential for toxicity.

____ 34. Fluoroquinolones and aminoglycosides were developed in response to increasing microorganism antibiotic drug resistance.

____ 35. Fluoroquinolones are bacteriostatic.

____ 36. Cipro is available in ophthalmic form as well as oral.

____ 37. All fluoroquinolones can cause the rupture of a tendon.

____ 38. Aminoglycosides are bacteriocidal.

____ 39. Aminoglycosides inhibit protein synthesis.

____ 40. Aminoglycosides are primarily used to treat infections caused by gram-negative microorganisms.

____ 41. Nephrotoxicity produced by aminoglycosides is irreversible.

____ 42. Ototoxicity produced by aminoglycoside therapy may occur during drug therapy or after the drug is discontinued.

____ 43. Aminoglycoside therapy is contraindicated in patients with Parkinsonism.

____ 44. When an aminoglycoside is being used, the patient's respiratory rate must be monitored.

____ 45. Fluoroquinolones may be given orally, parenterally, or intramuscularly.

____ 46. Any complaints from a patient receiving fluoroquinolone or aminoglycoside therapy should be reported.

VII. MULTIPLE CHOICE

Circle the letter of the best answer.

1. Which of the following sulfonamides are used to treat second- and third-degree burns?

   a. sulfisoxazole
   b. sulfasalazine
   c. sulfamethoxazole
   d. sulfamylon
   e. sulfamethizole

2. Sulfonamides can produce which of the following adverse reactions?

   a. Crystalluria
   b. Hypersensitivity reactions
   c. Anorexia
   d. Hematological changes
   e. All of the above

3. The most frequent adverse reaction seen with mafenide is ____.

   a. stomatitis
   b. burning sensation or pain
   c. fever
   d. increased appetite
   e. lesions on the skin at the injection site

4. The bacteriostatic activity of sulfonamides is due to the sulfonamides' ____.

   a. activity against the cell wall
   b. activity that inhibits metabolism
   c. overstimulation of cell growth
   d. antagonism to para-aminobenzoic acid
   e. Both a and c

5. When a sulfonamide is given with chlorprop-amide, the sulfonamide may ____.

   a. decrease the use of glucose
   b. increase the possibility of a hypoglycemic reaction
   c. lose its bacteriostatic ability
   d. increase its effectiveness
   e. None of the above

6. Sulfonamides are generally administered ____.

   a. on an empty stomach
   b. with a full glass of water
   c. with acidic fruit juices
   d. with milk or milk products
   e. Both a and b

7. Amoxicillin is an example of a(n) ____ penicillin.

   a. natural
   b. penicillinase-resistant
   c. amino

   d. extended-spectrum
   e. None of the above

8. Examples of beta-lactamase inhibitors are all of the following except ____.

   a. tazobactam
   b. clavulanic acid
   c. sulbactam
   d. All of the answers are beta-lactamase inhibitors

9. Penicillins may be effective against which of the following types of bacteria?

   a. Gonococci
   b. Staphylococci
   c. Streptococci
   d. Pneumococci
   e. All of the above

10. Pseudomembranous colitis is ____.

    a. a common type of fungal superinfection
    b. a common type of bacterial superinfection
    c. a common type of viral superinfection
    d. caused by an overgrowth of Clostridium difficile
    e. Both b and d

11. Intramuscular penicillin injections can cause ana-phylactic reactions that are most likely to occur ____.

    a. in 4 to 6 days
    b. within 30 minutes
    c. in 4 to 6 weeks
    d. only after multiple injections
    e. None of the above

12. Patients experiencing a dermatological reaction as the result of use of penicillin may ____.

    a. need to continue using the drug if the reaction is mild
    b. be prescribed an antihistamine
    c. need to use an antipyretic cream
    d. need to report this reaction to the health care provider
    e. All of the above

13. A first-generation cephalosporin would be more useful against ____.

    a. gram-negative organisms
    b. gram-positive organisms
    c. both gram-negative and gram-positive organisms
    d. fungal infections
    e. viral infections only

14. The most common adverse reaction of cephalo-sporins is ____.

    a. gastrointestinal disturbances
    b. visual disturbances
    c. diabetes
    d. sore throat
    e. ototoxicity

15. Patients receiving cephalosporin therapy should be closely monitored for ____.

    a. anemia
    b. nephrotoxicity
    c. signs of bacterial or fungal superinfections
    d. hypersensitivity reactions
    e. All of the above

16. An elderly patient receiving cephalosporin therapy who has existing renal impairment would prob-ably need ____.

    a. a higher dosage of drug and regular liver profile tests
    b. the same dosage of drug as a healthy patient and blood glucose monitoring
    c. a lower dosage of the drug and blood creati-nine level monitoring
    d. a higher dosage of the drug and blood glucose monitoring
    e. a lower dosage of the drug and regular liver profile tests

17. Which of the following is not an example of a tet-racycline?

    a. Vibramycin
    b. Tetracycline
    c. Doxycycline
    d. Clarithromycin
    e. Minocycline

18. Which of the following is an example of a macro-lide?

    a. erythromycin
    b. lincomycin
    c. clindamycin
    d. doxycycline

19. Clindamycin is an example of a ____.

    a. tetracycline
    b. macrolide
    c. cephalosporin
    d. penicillin
    e. lincosamide

20. Tetracyclines are used to treat ____.

    a. gram-negative and gram-positive microorgan-isms
    b. rickettsial infections
    c. intestinal amebiasis

    d. uncomplicated *Chlamydia trachomatis* infections
    e. All of the above

21. Tetracyclines are not given to children younger than 9 years of age unless absolutely necessary because ____.

    a. it retards their growth
    b. it may cause permanent yellow-gray-brown dis-coloration of their teeth
    c. it is too nephrotoxic for children
    d. it causes severe gastrointestinal upset
    e. of Stevens-Johnson syndrome

22. Macrolides act by ____.

    a. binding to cell membranes
    b. causing changes in protein function
    c. inhibiting bacterial replication
    d. Both a and b
    e. Both b and c

23. Macrolides should not be taken with ____.

    a. clindamycin
    b. lincomycin
    c. chloramphenicol
    d. None of the above
    e. Answers a, b, and c

24. Lincosamides are contraindicated in patients with ____.

    a. hypersensitivity
    b. minor bacterial infections
    c. minor viral infections
    d. infancy and lactation
    e. All of the above

25. When used with neuromuscular blocking drugs, lincosamides can enhance their effect and possibly lead to ____.

    a. severe tachycardia
    b. profound respiratory depression
    c. moderate respiratory stimulation
    d. urinary retention
    e. None of the above

26. Which of the following macrolides may be given without regard to meals?

    a. erythromycin
    b. clarithromycin
    c. azithromycin
    d. All of the above
    e. Both a and b

27. Fluoroquinolones are used to treat ____ infections.

    a. lower respiratory tract
    b. skin
    c. urinary tract
    d. sexually transmitted
    e. All of the above

28. ____ is an oral aminoglycoside used preoperatively to suppress gastrointestinal bacteria.
    a. kanamycin sulfate
    b. cipro
    c. penicillin G
    d. Both a and c
    e. Answers a, b, and c

29. ____ is used orally in the management of hepatic coma.
    a. amikacin
    b. paromomycin
    c. gentamicin
    d. tobramycin
    e. streptomycin

30. ____ produced by aminoglycoside therapy is(are) most often permanent.
    a. Liver damage
    b. Nephrotoxicity
    c. Visual disturbances
    d. Ototoxicity
    e. Both a and c

31. Mrs. P. has been taking an aminoglycoside and reports that her fingers are tingling. This may be indicative of ____.
    a. respiratory difficulties
    b. neurotoxicity
    c. nephrotoxicity
    d. hypersensitivity reactions
    e. None of the above

32. Auditory changes in patients taking an aminoglycoside may be ____.
    a. bilateral
    b. irreversible
    c. partial
    d. total
    e. All of the above

33. ____ are the only aminoglycosides that cannot be given either intravenously or intramuscularly.
    a. paromomycin and neomycin
    b. ampicillin and piperacillin
    c. cefprozil and cefuroxime
    d. neomycin and trimethoprim
    e. None of the above

34. Patient education about fluoroquinolone or aminoglycoside therapy is important because it ____.
    a. encourages compliance
    b. relieves anxiety
    c. promotes the desired result
    d. Both a and c
    e. Answers a, b, and c

VIII. RECALL FACTS

Indicate which of the following statements are facts with an F. If the statement is not a fact, leave the line blank.

ABOUT PSEUDOMEMBRANOUS COLITIS

____ 1. Is a common bacterial superinfection

____ 2. Is a potentially life-threatening problem

____ 3. Can also cause candidiasis

____ 4. Only occurs with extended drug use

____ 5. Is caused by an overgrowth of *C. difficile*

____ 6. Is easy to treat

____ 7. Has symptoms like diarrhea with blood and mucus

____ 8. Usually requires immediate discontinuation of the antibiotic

____ 9. May occur 4 to 9 days after treatment with penicillin

____ 10. May occur as long as 6 weeks after discontinuing the drug

ABOUT CEPHALOSPORINS

____ 1. Are classified as Pregnancy Category B drugs

____ 2. When taken with oral anticoagulants, the risk of bleeding decreases.

____ 3. Is safe to use alcohol during therapy

____ 4. When taken with aminoglycosides, the risk of nephrotoxicity increases.

____ 5. When alcohol is consumed, a disulfiram-like reaction may occur.

____ 6. Should be taken around the clock to maintain blood levels

____ 7. May be taken with food

____ 8. Examples are cefdinir, cefuroxime, and cefpodoxime

ABOUT TETRACYCLINE INTERACTIONS

___ 1. Counteract the action of aminoglycosides

___ 2. May decrease the effect of oral contraceptives

___ 3. May increase the effect of oral anticoagulants

___ 4. May increase the risk of digitalis toxicity

___ 5. Increase the effectiveness of cephalosporins

___ 6. May reduce insulin requirements

ABOUT FLUOROQUINOLONE INTERACTIONS

___ 1. Can increase the effects of oral anticoagulants

___ 2. Can increase serum theophylline levels

___ 3. Can increase cimetidine levels

___ 4. Antacids, iron salts, or zinc will increase absorption of fluoroquinolones.

___ 5. May increase risk of seizure with nonsteroidal anti-inflammatory drugs

___ 6. Increased risk of severe cardiac arrhythmias when given with procainamide

IX. FILL IN THE BLANKS

Fill in the blanks using words from the list below.

bacteriostatic	decrease	sulfonamides	alcoholic beverages	beta-lactamase
stop	increase	silver sulfadiazine	cephalosporins	urine output
penicillinase	bacteriocidal	parenteral	myasthenia gravis	minocycline
cephalosporins	oral	bacteriostatic	impair	liver disease
hour	DNA	nephrotoxicity		

1. Sulfonamides are primarily _____.

2. _____ may produce hematological changes such as agranulocytosis, thrombocytopenia, aplastic anemia, or leukopenia.

3. Any sign of leukopenia or thrombocytopenia in patients taking sulfonamides should be reported immediately because this is an indication to _____ drug therapy.

4. Patients with burns being treated with _____ should have the area inspected every 1 to 2 hours.

5. _____ is an enzyme produced by certain bacteria that inactivates penicillin.

6. The enzyme _____ is produced by certain bacteria and is able to destroy a component of penicillin.

7. Anaphylactic shock occurs more frequently after _____ use but can occur with _____ use.

8. The progression from first- to third-generation cephalosporin shows a(n) _____ in sensitivity to gram-negative organisms and a(n) _____ in sensitivity to gram-positive organisms.

9. An early sign of nephrotoxicity caused by the use of cephalosporins may be a decreased _____.

10. In patients who have a history of allergies to penicillins, the _____ are contraindicated.

11. Macrolides may be _____ or _____.

12. _____ is the tetracycline least likely to cause a photosensitivity reaction.

13. Antacids containing aluminum, zinc, magnesium, or bismuth salts or foods high in calcium _____ absorption of tetracyclines.

14. Macrolides are contraindicated in patients with preexisting _____.

15. The neuromuscular blocking action of lincosamides poses a danger to patients with

_____.

16. A patient with an elevated temperature who is taking a tetracycline, macrolide, or lincosamide should be monitored every _____ until the temperature returns to normal.

17. Fluoroquinolones act by interfering with an enzyme needed by the bacteria for _____ synthesis.

18. A patient taking an aminoglycoside with a urinary output of less than 750 ml/day may be at risk for

_____.

19. A patient receiving aminoglycoside or fluoroquinolone therapy should be cautioned against the use of _____ during therapy.

X. LIST

List the requested number of items.

1. List three bacteria that cause urinary tract infections that sulfonamides are often used to control.

   a. _____

   b. _____

   c. _____

2. List five signs of Stevens-Johnson syndrome.

   a. _____

   b. _____

   c. _____

   d. _____

   e. _____

3. List the four groups of penicillins.

   a. _____

   b. _____

   c. _____

   d. _____

4. List five types of infections that penicillins may be used to treat.

   a. _____

   b. _____

   c. _____

   d. _____

   e. _____

5. List five adverse reactions of penicillins.

   a. _____

   b. _____

   c. _____

   d. _____

   e. _____

6. List six infectious organisms that cephalosporins may be used to treat.

   a. _____

   b. _____

   c. _____

   d. _____

   e. _____

   f. _____

7. List five adverse reactions of lincosamides.

   a. _____

   b. _____

   c. _____

   d. _____

   e. _____

8. List five products that should not be taken with tetracyclines.

   a. _____

   b. _____

   c. _____

   d. _____

   e. _____

9. List five examples of fluoroquinolones.

   a. _____

   b. _____

   c. _____

   d. _____

   e. _____

10. List five potential adverse reactions of aminoglycosides.

    a. _____

    b. _____

   c. _____

   d. _____

   e. _____

11. List five aminoglycosides that are Pregnancy Category D drugs.

    a. _____

    b. _____

    c. _____

    d. _____

    e. _____

12. List three fluoroquinolones that may be given intravenously.

    a. _____

    b. _____

    c. _____

XI. CLINICAL APPLICATIONS

1. Miss P., age 83, cannot remember if she is allergic to penicillin. What symptoms might you ask her about to help determine if she has had a hypersensitivity reaction to these drugs in the past?

2. Mrs. R. has been prescribed a cephalosporin for her infection. She has been advised to be on the alert for a superinfection but does not know what the symptoms of this are. Explain to Mrs. R. and her family what she should look for.

XII. CASE STUDY

Mr. A. has been put on the aminoglycoside paromomycin for intestinal amebiasis. Mr. A. and his family are asking questions about this drug and what they can expect while he is being treated.

1. All of the following are adverse reactions seen with aminoglycosides except _____.

   a. nephrotoxicity
   b. ototoxicity
   c. neurotoxicity
   d. long QT syndrome

2. Oral aminoglycosides are usually given _____.

   a. before meals
   b. after meals
   c. without regard to meals
   d. with milk

3. Which of the following is true about fluid intake while taking an aminoglycoside?

   a. The patient must drink 6 to 8 glasses of water daily.
   b. Each dose should be taken with a full glass of water.
   c. Fluid intake must be decreased while on this drug.
   d. Both a and b
   e. None of the above

36

Antimycobacterial Drugs

I. MATCH THE FOLLOWING

Match the term from Column A with the correct definition from Column B.

COLUMN A

_____ 1. Anaphylactoid reaction

_____ 2. Antitubercular drugs

_____ 3. Leprosy

_____ 4. *Mycobacterium leprae*

_____ 5. *Mycobacterium tuberculosis*

_____ 6. Tuberculosis

COLUMN B

A. A disease caused by *Mycobacterium tuberculosis*

B. The bacteria that cause leprosy

C. A chronic, communicable disease spread by prolonged intimate contact with an infected person.

D. The bacteria that cause tuberculosis.

E. Unusual or exaggerated allergic reaction.

F. Drugs used to treat active causes of tuberculosis.

II. MATCH THE FOLLOWING

Match the generic name of antitubercular or leprostatic from Column A with the correct trade name from Column B.

COLUMN A

_____ 1. aminosalicylate

_____ 2. ethambutol

_____ 3. ethionamide

_____ 4. capreomycin

_____ 5. rifabutin

_____ 6. cycloserine

_____ 7. rifapentine

_____ 8. rifampin

_____ 9. dapsone

COLUMN B

A. Priftin

B. Seromycin

C. Capastat Sulfate

D. Paser

E. Rifadin

F. Myambutol

G. Mycobutin

H. Aczone

I. Trecator

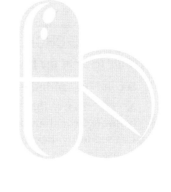

III. MATCH THE FOLLOWING

Match the trade name from Column A with the drug category from Column B. You may use an answer more than once.

COLUMN A

____ 1. Capastat sulfate

____ 2. Myambutol

____ 3. Aczone

____ 4. INH

____ 5. Mycobutin

____ 6. Rifadin

____ 7. Paser

____ 8. Priftin

____ 9. Trecator

____ 10. Seromycin

COLUMN B

A. Antitubercular—first-line

B. Antitubercular—second-line

C. Leprostatic

IV. TRUE OR FALSE

Indicate whether each statement is True (T) or False (F).

____ 1. Antitubercular drug therapy can cure a patient with tuberculosis.

____ 2. Isoniazid is the only bactericidal antitubercular drug.

____ 3. Antitubercular drugs work by inhibiting bacterial cell wall synthesis.

____ 4. Vision changes related to ethambutol are usually reversible if the drug is discontinued as soon as symptoms appear.

____ 5. Hepatitis, a potential adverse reaction of isoniazid therapy, only occurs during treatment.

____ 6. Rifampin may cause a reddish orange discoloration of body fluids.

____ 7. Isoniazid and rifampin used concurrently may result in a higher risk of hepatotoxicity than when either drug is used alone.

____ 8. Directly observed therapy for treatment of tuberculosis may be necessary to assure compliance with the treatment regimen.

____ 9. Leprostatic drugs cure leprosy.

____ 10. Clofazimine and dapsone have no significant drug–drug interactions.

V. MULTIPLE CHOICE

Circle the letter of the best answer.

1. Second-line antitubercular drugs are ____.
   a. less effective than primary drugs
   b. more toxic than primary drugs
   c. used to treat extrapulmonary tuberculosis
   d. used to treat drug-resistant tuberculosis
   e. All of the above

2. Isoniazid's primary use is ____.
   a. part of second-line therapy
   b. preventive therapy against tuberculosis
   c. part of primary drug therapy
   d. for treatment of children with tuberculosis
   e. for treating pregnant women with tuberculosis

3. Re-treatment regimens for tuberculosis therapy include all the following drugs except ____.
   a. capreomycin
   b. cycloserine
   c. isoniazid
   d. aminosalicylic acid

4. Patients taking isoniazid should ____.
   a. not eat foods with tyramine
   b. not consume alcohol
   c. not use products with aluminum salts
   d. have liver enzyme test
   e. All of the above

5. ____ is the principal adverse reaction of pyrazin-amide use.

    a. Optic neuritis
    b. Hepatotoxicity
    c. Kidney failure
    d. Hypertension
    e. Asthma

6. Streptomycin may cause ____.

    a. permanent hearing loss
    b. fetal harm
    c. hepatotoxicity
    d. Both a and b
    e. Both b and c

7. Which of the following antitubercular drugs is given daily as an intramuscular injection?

    a. rifabutin
    b. rifampin

    c. streptomycin
    d. ethambutol
    e. pyrazinamide

8. Which of the following antitubercular drugs may cause the patient's urine, feces, or saliva to turn reddish orange?

    a. ethambutol
    b. isoniazid
    c. rifampin
    d. Both a and c
    e. None of the above

9. Dapsone is used to treat ____.

    a. dermatitis
    b. leprosy
    c. tuberculosis
    d. All of the above (options a–c are correct)
    e. Both a and b

VI. RECALL FACTS

Indicate which of the following statements are facts with an F. If the statement is not a fact, leave the line blank.

ABOUT ANTITUBERCULAR DRUGS

____ 1. Most antitubercular drugs are bacteriostatic.

____ 2. Isoniazid is never used alone.

____ 3. The standard treatment for tuberculosis is divided into two phases.

____ 4. At times, treatment fails because of noncompliance.

____ 5. Optic neuritis has occurred in some patients receiving ethambutol.

____ 6. Older adults are particularly susceptible to a potentially fatal hepatitis when taking isoniazid.

VII. FILL IN THE BLANKS

Fill in the blanks using words from the list below.

acute gout	bacteriostatic	dapsone	hemolytic reactions
pyrazinamide	bactericidal	dapsone	drug-related hepatitis
13	digoxin	optic neuritis	ethambutol

1. The CDC treatment recommendations for tuberculosis in areas of low incidence for the initial phase include the use of rifampin, isoniazid, _____, and _____ for a minimum of 2 months.

2. _____ is an adverse reaction of ethambutol, which appears to be related to the dose given and the duration of treatment.

3. Pyrazinamide is contraindicated in patients with _____ and severe liver damage.

4. _____ can be used to treat leprosy.

5. Dapsone is _____ and _____ against *M. leprae.*

6. Significant amounts of _____ are excreted in breast milk and can cause _____ in neonates.

7. Daily consumption of alcohol when taking isoniazid may result in a higher incidence of _____.

8. Ethambutol is not recommended for children younger than _____ years.

9. Serum concentration of _____ may be decreased by rifampin.

VIII. LIST

List the requested number of items.

1. List four drugs that can be used in the initial phase of standard treatment for tuberculosis.

    a. _____

    b. _____

    c. _____

    d. _____

2. List six prophylactic uses of isoniazid.

    a. _____

    b. _____

    c. _____

    d. _____

    e. _____

    f. _____

3. List four drugs included in regimens most often used for retreatment of tuberculosis.

    a. _____

    b. _____

    c. _____

    d. _____

4. List five adverse reactions to isoniazid.

    a. _____

    b. _____

    c. _____

    d. _____

    e. _____

IX. CLINICAL APPLICATIONS

1. Mr. X., age 73, has recently been diagnosed with tuberculosis. As his health status is evaluated, the care team must be aware of the fact that other organs could be affected by the organism in addition to the lungs. What organs may need to be evaluated? Who should be treated in addition to Mr. X.?

X. CASE STUDY

Mrs. J. has been placed on ethambutol for her tuberculosis. This drug has quite a few potential adverse reactions associated with it that Mrs. J. and her health care provider need to be aware of.

1. Optic neuritis may occur with ethambutol usage. All of the following are true about optic neuritis and ethambutol except:

    a. Optic neuritis causes a decrease in visual acuity.
    b. Changes in color perception occur with optic neuritis.
    c. The presence of optic neuritis is in no way related to the dose of ethambutol given.
    d. The presence of optic neuritis is related to the duration of treatment.
    e. This adverse reaction usually disappears when the drug is discontinued.

2. Other adverse reactions of the drug are _____.

    a. dermatitis
    b. pruritus
    c. anaphylactoid reaction
    d. joint pain
    e. All of the above
    f. Both a and b

3. Psychic disturbances may occur while on this drug. The patient must be monitored for _____.

    a. depression
    b. withdrawal
    c. personality changes
    d. All of the above
    e. None of the above

37

Antiviral, Antiretroviral, and Antifungal Drugs

I. MATCH THE FOLLOWING

Match the term from Column A with the correct definition from Column B.

COLUMN A

____ 1. Fungicidal

____ 2. Mycotic infection

____ 3. Onychomycosis

____ 4. Tinea cruris

____ 5. Viral load

COLUMN B

A. Jock itch

B. A superficial or deep infection caused by a fungi disease in humans that may be yeast-like or mold-like

C. Able to destroy fungi

D. Nail fungus condition

E. The blood level of HIV viral RNA; used for monitoring the course of AIDS

II. MATCH THE FOLLOWING

Match the generic antiviral drug from Column A with the correct trade name from Column B.

COLUMN A

____ 1. acyclovir

____ 2. cidofovir

____ 3. valganciclovir

____ 4. adefovir

____ 5. zanamivir

____ 6. boceprevir

____ 7. valacyclovir

____ 8. oseltamivir

____ 9. ganciclovir

____ 10. famciclovir

____ 11. amantadine

____ 12. rimantadine

____ 13. ribavirin

____ 14. telaprevir

____ 15. entecavir

COLUMN B

A. Cytovene

B. Tamiflu

C. Flumadine

D. Copegus

E. Incivek

F. Hepsera

G. Valcyte

H. Symmetrel

I. Zovirax

J. Valtrex

K. Baraclude

L. Famvir

M. Victrelis

N. Relenza

O. Vistide

III. MATCH THE FOLLOWING

Match the generic antifungal drug from Column A with the correct trade name from Column B.

COLUMN A

_____ 1. itraconazole

_____ 2. ketoconazole

_____ 3. fluconazole

_____ 4. amphotericin B

_____ 5. flucytosine (5-FC)

_____ 6. caspofungin acetate

_____ 7. griseofulvin microsize

_____ 8. micafungin

COLUMN B

A. Diflucan

B. Ancobon

C. Nizoral

D. Sporanox

E. Grifulvin V

F. Cancidas

G. Mycamine

H. Abelcet

IV. MATCH THE FOLLOWING

Match the generic topical antifungal drug from Column A with the correct trade name from Column B.

COLUMN A

_____ 1. naftifine

_____ 2. undecylenic acid

_____ 3. miconazole

_____ 4. clotrimazole

_____ 5. nystatin

_____ 6. tolnaftate

_____ 7. butenafine

_____ 8. ciclopirox

COLUMN B

A. Lotrimin

B. Loprox

C. Mentax

D. Tinactin

E. Naftin

F. Cruex

G. Nyamyc

H. Monistat

V. MATCH THE FOLLOWING

Match the trade name from Column A with the type of anti-infective from Column B. You may use an answer more than once.

COLUMN A

_____ 1. Naftin

_____ 2. Abelcet

_____ 3. Mentax

_____ 4. Nizoral

_____ 5. Monistat-1

_____ 6. Zovirax

_____ 7. Victrelis

_____ 8. Desenex

_____ 9. Famvir

_____ 10. Vfend

_____ 11. Cytovene

_____ 12. Terazol

_____ 13. Lotrimin AF

_____ 14. Ertaczo

COLUMN B

A. Antiviral

B. Antifungal, oral or parenteral

C. Topical antifungal

D. Vaginal antifungal

VI. MATCH THE FOLLOWING

Match the antiviral trade name from Column A with the correct use from Column B. You may use an answer more than once.

COLUMN A

____ 1. Valcyte

____ 2. Cytovene

____ 3. Famvir

____ 4. Vistide

____ 5. Virazole

____ 6. Tamiflu

____ 7. Relenza

____ 8. Hespera

____ 9. Zovirax

____ 10. Valtrex

____ 11. Victrelis

____ 12. Baraclude

____ 13. Flumadine

____ 14. Incivek

COLUMN B

A. Acute herpes zoster

B. Severe lower respiratory tract infection

C. Influenza virus

D. Chronic hepatitis B

E. HSV type 2

F. CMV retinitis

G. Chronic hepatitis C

H. Influenza A virus

VII. MATCH THE FOLLOWING

Match the fungicide from Column A with the mode of action from Column B. You may use an answer more than once or not at all.

COLUMN A

____ 1. Diflucan

____ 2. Lotrimin

____ 3. Grifulvin-V

____ 4. Nizoral

____ 5. Monistat

____ 6. Ancobon

____ 7. Amphotec

COLUMN B

A. Not clearly understood

B. Is deposited in keratin precursor cells that are then lost and replaced by uninfected cells

C. Affects cell membrane

D. Causes depletion of sterols

E. Related to concentration in body tissues

F. Causes cells to die

G. Binds with phospholipids in fungal cell membrane increasing permeability of the cell

VIII. MATCH THE FOLLOWING

Match the generic antiviral drug from Column A with the correct trade name from Column B.

COLUMN A

____ 1. maraviroc

____ 2. abacavir

____ 3. atazanavir

____ 4. ritonavir

____ 5. enfuvirtide

____ 6. emtricitabine

____ 7. efavirenz

____ 8. zidovudine

COLUMN B

A. Ziagen

B. Retrovir

C. Selzentry

D. Fuzeon

E. Norvir

F. Sustiva

G. Emtriva

H. Reyataz

IX. TRUE OR FALSE

Indicate whether each statement is True (T) or False (F).

_____ 1. Most antiviral drugs act by inhibiting viral DNA or RNA replication in the virus.

_____ 2. All antiviral drugs are contraindicated in patients with congestive heart failure and during lactation.

_____ 3. A rash at the site of application is a normal reaction to a topical antiviral drug.

_____ 4. Acyclovir, in any form of administration, has no precautions; it is safe for everyone to use.

_____ 5. Zanamivir can cause serious adverse reactions such as bronchospasm, which can lead to death.

_____ 6. A mycotic infection is caused by a plant that contains chlorophyll.

_____ 7. Deep mycotic infections are among the easiest to treat because of their limited location.

_____ 8. Topical antifungal drugs generally cause few adverse reactions.

_____ 9. Some adverse reactions of amphotericin B may be lessened by the use of aspirin, antihistamines, or antiemetics.

_____ 10. Amphotericin B may be nephrotoxic.

_____ 11. Fluconazole can alter liver function.

_____ 12. Gastrointestinal distress is rarely a problem with flucytosine use.

_____ 13. Patients taking griseofulvin should avoid exposure to direct sunlight.

_____ 14. Patients may develop hepatitis during itraconazole use.

_____ 15. Few patients can tolerate ketoconazole without severe adverse reactions.

_____ 16. Tea tree oil is an effective antifungal that is used to relieve and control the symptoms of tinea pedis.

X. MULTIPLE CHOICE

Circle the letter of the best answer.

1. Antiviral drugs may be given as _____.
   a. topical drugs
   b. systemic drugs
   c. oral drugs
   d. intravenous drugs
   e. All of the above

2. The most common adverse reaction(s) of antiviral drugs that are administered systemically is (are) _____.
   a. visual disturbances
   b. gastrointestinal disturbances
   c. reproductive difficulties
   d. CNS depression
   e. musculoskeletal twitching

3. The antiviral drug _____ is a Pregnancy Category X drug.
   a. ribavirin
   b. amprenavir
   c. ganciclovir
   d. imiquimod
   e. ritonavir

4. Acyclovir _____.
   a. can be used orally, topically, or parenterally
   b. can cause crystalluria if adequate hydration is not maintained
   c. treatment should begin as soon as symptoms of herpes simplex appear
   d. can be given without regard to food
   e. All of the above

5. Amantadine is used with caution in all of the following conditions except _____.
   a. seizure disorders
   b. psychiatric problems
   c. emphysema
   d. kidney impairment
   e. cardiac disease

6. Amantadine patients should be monitored for which of the following?
   a. Mood changes
   b. Thrombocytopenia
   c. Liver function
   d. Cardiac output
   e. Polycythemia

7. Amantadine is used _____.
   a. to treat HIV
   b. for herpes simplex viral infections
   c. to manage the extrapyramidal effects of drugs used to treat parkinsonism
   d. for the prevention and treatment of respiratory tract illness caused by influenza type A virus
   e. Both c and d

8. Ribavirin ____.
   a. is a Pregnancy Category X drug
   b. can cause worsening of respiratory status
   c. is safe to use in patients with COPD
   d. can antagonize the action of zidovudine
   e. All of the above, except c

9. Zidovudine ____.
   a. should be used with caution in patients with bone marrow depression
   b. interacts with methadone
   c. interacts with doxorubicin
   d. Both a and b
   e. Answers a, b, and c

10. Lemon balm (*Melissa officinalis*) traditionally has been used ____.
    a. for Graves disease
    b. as a sedative
    c. as an antispasmodic
    d. as an antiviral agent
    e. All of the above

11. Fungal infections may be ____.
    a. superficial
    b. systemic
    c. intradermal
    d. Both a and b
    e. Both b and c

12. All of the following are examples of superficial mycotic infections except:
    a. Hydatid disease
    b. Onychomycosis
    c. Tinea cruris
    d. Tinea pedis
    e. Tinea corporis

13. Amphotericin B ____.
    a. is given parenterally
    b. is given for several months
    c. use often results in serious reactions
    d. is reserved for serious and potentially life-threatening fungal infections
    e. All of the above

14. All of the following statements about amphotericin B are true except:
    a. Amphotericin B is given only under close supervision in the hospital.
    b. Amphotericin B can cause severe bone marrow depression.
    c. When given with corticosteroids, amphotericin B may cause hyperkalemia.

    d. Amphotericin B is a Pregnancy Category B drug and is used cautiously during lactation.
    e. Amphotericin B is used cautiously in patients with renal dysfunction or electrolyte imbalances.

15. Fluconazole ____.
    a. may decrease the metabolism of phenytoin and warfarin
    b. may cause an increased effect of an oral hypoglycemic
    c. may be given orally or intravenously
    d. is considered to be a Pregnancy Category B drug
    e. All of the above, except d

16. Flucytosine may have ____ as (an) adverse reaction(s).
    a. anemia
    b. leukopenia
    c. thrombocytopenia
    d. All of the above
    e. Both a and c

17. A patient taking griseofulvin may have a decreased effect of the drug when which of the following drugs are taken concurrently?
    a. Warfarin
    b. Barbiturate
    c. Oral contraceptives
    d. Salicylate concentrations
    e. All of the above

18. Itraconazole ____.
    a. can be given orally with food to increase absorption
    b. can be used topically
    c. is often diluted with saline for intravenous infusion
    d. should be given with milk
    e. is often given on an empty stomach to increase absorption

19. Ketoconazole ____.
    a. is commonly given with food
    b. is commonly given with antacids, anticholinergics, or histamine blockers
    c. usually causes severe adverse reactions
    d. is a Pregnancy Category B drug
    e. All of the above

20. Miconazole ____.
    a. is used to treat vulvovaginal fungal infections
    b. is used during the first trimester only when essential
    c. may cause irritation, sensitization, or vulvovaginal burning
    d. is usually self-administered on an outpatient basis
    e. All of the above

21. Which of the following herbs have been identified as being effective against tinea pedis?
    a. Oral ingestion of garlic tablets
    b. 10% tea tree oil cream
    c. 0.4% ajoene cream
    d. Both b and c
    e. All of the above

22. Zidovudine interacts with all of the following except _____.
    a. NSAIDs
    b. doxorubicin
    c. methadone
    d. probenecid

23. Patients receiving antiviral drugs for human immunodeficiency infections may continue to have opportunistic infections and should be closely monitored for signs of infection such as _____.
    a. fever (even low-grade)
    b. nausea
    c. malaise
    d. sore throat
    e. lethargy
    f. All of the above, except b

XI. RECALL FACTS

Indicate which of the following statements are facts with an F. If the statement is not a fact, leave the line blank.

ABOUT EDUCATING THE PATIENT AND FAMILY ABOUT ANTIVIRAL DRUGS

_____ 1. These drugs cure viral infections.

_____ 2. These drugs should decrease the symptoms of viral infections.

_____ 3. A missed dose should not be doubled at the next dosage time.

_____ 4. Symptoms of infection should be reported.

_____ 5. It is common practice to stop the medication once the patient feels better.

_____ 6. Signs of pancreatitis need to be reported immediately.

_____ 7. Peripheral neuropathy is to be expected and tolerated by the patient.

ABOUT GENERAL PATIENT MANAGEMENT ISSUES WITH ANTIFUNGAL DRUGS

_____ 1. Oral and parenteral drug routes require patient observation every 2 to 4 hours for adverse reactions.

_____ 2. Topical antifungal drug use should be monitored weekly.

_____ 3. Antifungal drug therapy may require weeks to months.

_____ 4. Drugs that are potentially toxic to the kidneys only require fluid monitoring.

_____ 5. Serum creatinine and blood urea nitrogen levels should be checked frequently during therapy.

_____ 6. Gloves should be used when caring for open lesions.

XII. FILL IN THE BLANKS

Fill in the blanks using words from the list below.

zidovudine	*Candida albicans*	inhalation	fungus
topical	2	amphotericin B	kidney damage
diabetes	oral thrush	fluconazole hepatotoxicity	flucytosine

1. _____ administration of antiviral drugs can cause transient burning, stinging, and pruritus as adverse reactions.

2. Ribavirin is given by _____.

3. Zanamivir drug therapy should be started within _____ days' onset of flu symptoms.

4. _____ drug therapy can cause severe hepatomegaly and bone marrow depression.

5. A(n) _____ is a colorless plant that lacks chlorophyll.

6. _____ commonly causes yeast infections in women.

7. _____ is the most effective drug available for the treatment of most systemic fungal infections.

8. _____ is the most serious adverse reaction of amphotericin B.

9. _____ may increase an older patient's risk of decreased renal and liver function.

10. Before therapy is begun with _____, the patient's hematological, electrolyte, and renal status are determined.

11. Griseofulvin can cause _____ to occur.

12. Itraconazole and ketoconazole use may cause _____.

13. Patients with recurrent or chronic cases of candidiasis who repeatedly are prescribed miconazole should be evaluated for _____.

XIII. LIST

List the requested number of items.

1. List seven uses of antiviral drugs.

   a. _____

   b. _____

   c. _____

   d. _____

   e. _____

   f. _____

   g. _____

2. List five drugs that when used concurrently with amantadine may increase its anticholinergic effects.

   a. _____

   b. _____

   c. _____

   d. _____

   e. _____

3. List five adverse reactions of amphotericin B.

   a. _____

   b. _____

   c. _____

   d. _____

   e. _____

4. List four drugs that interact with itraconazole and cause a decrease in the blood levels of itraconazole.

   a. _____

   b. _____

   c. _____

   d. _____

5. List four adverse reactions seen with maraviroc.

   a. _____

   b. _____

   c. _____

   d. _____

XIV. CLINICAL APPLICATIONS

1. Miss P has been diagnosed with a herpes simplex infection. She is to take the oral medication (Zovirax) for her treatment. Explain to Miss P what precautions she must follow while taking this medication.

XV. CASE STUDY

Mr. M. has been diagnosed with HIV and has been prescribed zidovudine. You are giving him instructions related to taking this drug and general information about antiretroviral drugs.

1. Zidovudine is a nucleoside/nucleotide analog reverse transcriptase inhibitor. How would you explain the action of this drug to Mr. M.?

   a. It blocks an enzyme involved with the virus's ability to multiply.
   b. It cures the disease.
   c. It leads to inhibited viral DNA growth.
   d. It prevents the HIV virus from entering the cells.

2. Key point(s) about antiretroviral drugs that the patient and family should know include(s) _____.

   a. antiretroviral drugs are not a cure for disease
   b. these drugs do not reduce the risk of transmitting HIV to others
   c. the medication should be taken exactly as prescribed
   d. doses should not be skipped or discontinued without direction from the health care provider
   e. All of the above.

3. Adverse reactions to zidovudine include all of the following except _____.

   a. lactic acidosis
   b. severe hepatomegaly
   c. peripheral neuropathy
   d. lipoatrophy

38

Antiparasitic Drugs

I. MATCH THE FOLLOWING

Match the term from Column A with the correct definition from Column B.

COLUMN A

___ 1. Anthelmintic

___ 2. Helminthiasis

___ 3. Parasite

___ 4. Amebiasis

___ 5. Helminths

___ 6. Cinchonism

COLUMN B

A. A group of symptoms associated with quinine

B. Invasion of the body by helminths

C. Drugs with actions against helminths

D. An organism that lives in or on another organism without contributing to the survival or well-being of the host

E. Worms

F. Invasion of the body by the ameba *Entamoeba histolytica*

II. MATCH THE FOLLOWING

Match the generic anthelmintic, antimalarial, or amebicide from Column A with the correct trade name from Column B.

COLUMN A

___ 1. metronidazole

___ 2. atovaquone and proguanil HCL

___ 3. pyrimethamine

___ 4. quinine

___ 5. chloroquine hydrochloride

___ 6. iodoquinol

___ 7. pyrantel

___ 8. praziquantel

___ 9. ivermectin

___ 10. albendazole

___ 11. artemether/lumefantrine

___ 12. hydroxychloroquine sulfate

___ 13. chloroquine phosphate

COLUMN B

A. Daraprim

B. Flagyl

C. Antiminth

D. Aralen

E. Biltricide

F. Malarone

G. Qualaquin

H. Stromectol

I. Aralen

J. Yodoxin

K. Plaquenil

L. Coartem

M. Albenza

III. MATCH THE FOLLOWING

Match the trade name from Column A with the type of anti-infective from Column B. You may use an answer more than once.

COLUMN A

____ 1. Antiminth
____ 2. Aralen
____ 3. Yodoxin
____ 4. Plaquenil
____ 5. Biltricide
____ 6. Malarone
____ 7. Vermox

COLUMN B

A. Anthelmintic
B. Antimalarial
C. Amebicide

IV. MATCH THE FOLLOWING

Match the trade name of the anthelmintic, antimalarial, or amebicide drug from Column A with the correct use from Column B. You may use an answer more than once.

COLUMN A

____ 1. Flagyl
____ 2. Malarone
____ 3. Albenza
____ 4. Aralen
____ 5. Plaquenil
____ 6. Daraprim
____ 7. quinine
____ 8. mebendazole
____ 9. Pin-X

COLUMN B

A. Hydatid disease
B. Treatment of intestinal amebiasis
C. Treatment of malaria
D. Prevention and treatment of malaria
E. Roundworm and pinworm
F. American hookworm, whipworm, pinworm, roundworm

V. MATCH THE FOLLOWING

Match the anthelmintic drug from Column A with the action from Column B.

COLUMN A

____ 1. albendazole
____ 2. mebendazole
____ 3. pyrantel
____ 4. ivermectin

COLUMN B

A. Interferes with the synthesis of the parasites microtubules
B. Blocks the uptake of glucose by the helminth
C. Leads to an increase in the permeability of the cell membrane to chloride ions with hyperpolarization of the nerve or muscle cell
D. Paralyzes the helminth

VI. TRUE OR FALSE

Indicate whether each statement is True (T) or False (F).

_____ 1. Albenza works by interfering with the synthesis of the parasite's microtubules.

_____ 2. The five anthelmintic drugs discussed in Chapter 38 are all Pregnancy Category B drugs.

_____ 3. Mebendazole can cause leukopenia or thrombocytopenia.

_____ 4. Diarrhea is a common adverse reaction of anthelmintic drugs.

_____ 5. Malaria is caused by the protozoan species *Anopheles*.

_____ 6. The symptoms of malaria appear when the sporozoites enter the person's bloodstream.

_____ 7. Aralen is only used in the treatment of malaria.

_____ 8. All antimalarial drugs work equally well in suppressing or treating all four of the *Plasmodium* species that cause malaria.

_____ 9. Chloroquine should be used with extreme caution in children.

_____ 10. Quinine is contraindicated in pregnant women and in patients with myasthenia gravis.

_____ 11. Visual disturbances observed in patients taking chloroquine have caused no long-term problems.

_____ 12. Amebicides kill amebas.

_____ 13. Extraintestinal amebiasis is more difficult to treat.

_____ 14. Rare but serious adverse reactions of paromomycin are nephrotoxicity and ototoxicity.

_____ 15. It is common practice to test immediate family members for amebiasis.

VII. MULTIPLE CHOICE

Circle the letter of the best answer.

1. All the following drugs are considered to be anthelmintic drugs except _____.

   a. albendazole
   b. praziquantel
   c. mebendazole
   d. pyrantel
   e. metronidazole

2. Which of the following anthelmintic drugs have been shown to cause embryotoxic and teratogenic effects in experimental animals?

   a. albendazole and pyrantel
   b. mebendazole and thiabendazole
   c. albendazole and mebendazole
   d. pyrantel and thiabendazole
   e. mebendazole and pyrantel

3. Which of the following anthelmintic drugs may be taken without regard to food?

   a. mebendazole
   b. thiabendazole
   c. albendazole
   d. pyrantel
   e. All of the drugs should be taken with food to increase absorption.

4. When chloroquine is used for prophylaxis, therapy should begin _____ weeks before exposure and continue for _____ weeks after exposure.

   a. 2, 6 to 8
   b. 4, 1 to 2
   c. 6, 2
   d. 6 to 8, 2
   e. 10, 10

5. A patient taking chloroquine may experience which of the following visual disturbances?

   a. Disturbed color vision
   b. Blurred vision
   c. Night blindness
   d. Diminished visual fields
   e. All of the above

6. Which of the following drugs are used to treat intestinal amebiasis?

   a. Aralen
   b. miconazole
   c. doxycycline
   d. Yodoxin
   e. pyrantel

7. All of the following drugs are used to treat amebiasis except _____.
   a. iodoquinol
   b. vibramycin
   c. metronidazole
   d. paromomycin
   e. chloroquine hydrochloride

8. Patients taking amebicides _____.
   a. may be at risk for dehydration
   b. should take the drug exactly as prescribed
   c. should wash hands immediately before eating or preparing food and after defecation
   d. may need to have stool specimens saved for laboratory analysis
   e. All of the above.

VIII. RECALL FACTS

Indicate which of the following statements are facts with an F. If the statement is not a fact, leave the line blank.

ABOUT ANTIMALARIAL DRUGS

____ 1. Chloroquine is used cautiously in patients with liver disease or bone marrow depression.

____ 2. Quinine can cause cinchonism at full therapeutic doses.

____ 3. Adverse reactions with quinine include diarrhea and abdominal cramps.

____ 4. Plasma levels of warfarin are increased when taking quinine.

____ 5. Absorption of artemether/lumefantrine is enhanced when taking with food.

____ 6. Antimalarial drugs interfere with the lifecycle of the plasmodium.

IX. FILL IN THE BLANKS

Fill in the blanks using words from the list below.

reduce	anthelmintic drugs	exactly	intestinal	delayed
cinchonism	acidify	antimalarial	pyrantel	Flagyl
iodoquinol	alcohol	bowel	amebiasis	C

1. The prime purpose of _____ is to kill the parasite.

2. Use of mebendazole with the hydantoins and carbamazepine may _____ plasma levels of mebendazole.

3. _____ and piperazine are antagonists and should not be given together.

4. _____ drugs interfere with the life cycle of the plasmodium, primarily when it is present in red blood cells.

5. Foods that _____ the urine may increase excretion and decrease the effectiveness of chloroquine.

6. The use of quinine can cause _____ at full therapeutic doses.

7. Quinine is a Pregnancy Category _____ drug.

8. Quinine absorption is _____ when taken with antacids containing aluminum.

9. Antimalarial drugs taken for suppression of malaria should be taken _____ as prescribed.

10. The two types of amebiasis are _____ and extraintestinal.

11. _____ is used to treat intestinal amebiasis.

12. _____ may interfere with thyroid function tests for as long as 6 months after therapy is discontinued.

13. Patients taking metronidazole must avoid _____ while undergoing treatment.

14. Paromomycin is given with caution to patients with _____ disease.

15. Patients with _____ may or may not be acutely ill and may require isolation procedures.

X. LIST

List the requested number of items.

1. List five examples of helminths.

   a. _____

   b. _____

   c. _____

   d. _____

   e. _____

2. List three precautions that should be taken by the health care worker when dealing with a patient who has a helminth infection.

   a. _____

   b. _____

   c. _____

3. List the four protozoans that can cause malaria.

   a. _____

   b. _____

   c. _____

   d. _____

4. List six adverse reactions of chloroquine.

   a. _____

   b. _____

   c. _____

   d. _____

   e. _____

   f. _____

5. List five symptoms of cinchonism.

   a. _____

   b. _____

   c. _____

   d. _____

   e. _____

XI. CLINICAL APPLICATIONS

1. Mrs. C's daughter, who is 17 years old, has been invited to participate in a school trip to an area that has malaria. The school nurse has sent a note home with the students that states that they must see their family physician soon to get started on the required medication for the trip. Explain to Mrs. C the key points about treatment with malaria drugs and why it is important for her daughter to take the medication exactly as prescribed.

XII. CASE STUDY

A 1-year-old child in the M. family has been diagnosed with amebiasis. He has been losing weight and has been suffering from frequent diarrhea. He has been put on the drug iodoquinal.

1. What further measures may be required related to discovery of this disease in a family?

   a. The health department may require investigation into the source of the infection.
   b. The water supply to the home may be analyzed.
   c. Immediate family members may be tested for amebiasis.
   d. All of the above.

2. What side effects may be seen with this drug?

   a. Nausea
   b. Vomiting
   c. Black tongue
   d. Paresthesias
   e. Both a and b

3. What is true related to the use of amebicides?

   a. The full course of treatment must be completed.
   b. The patient must follow the directions for taking the medication exactly as prescribed.
   c. The family must follow measures to control the spread of infection.
   d. Family members must wash hands immediately before eating or preparing food and after defecation.
   e. All of the above.

39

Miscellaneous Anti-Infectives

I. MATCH THE FOLLOWING

Match the term from Column A with the correct definition from Column B.

COLUMN A

_____ 1. Anaerobic

_____ 2. Trichomonas

_____ 3. Nosocomial pneumonia

_____ 4. Red Man Syndrome

_____ 5. Nephrotoxicity

_____ 6. Ototoxicity

COLUMN B

A. A parasitic protozoan

B. Able to live without oxygen

C. Hospital-acquired pneumonia

D. Severe adverse reaction to vancomycin

E. Damage to the organs of hearing; may occur with vancomycin

F. Damage to the kidneys; may occur with vancomycin

II. MATCH THE FOLLOWING

Match the generic name of the miscellaneous anti-infective from Column A with the correct trade name from Column B.

COLUMN A

_____ 1. linezolid

_____ 2. meropenem

_____ 3. metronidazole

_____ 4. pentamidine isoethionate

_____ 5. vancomycin

COLUMN B

A. Zyvox

B. Vancocin

C. Flagyl

D. Merrem

E. NebuPent

III. TRUE OR FALSE

Indicate whether each statement is True (T) or False (F).

_____ 1. Patients receiving oral chloramphenicol are often hospitalized.

_____ 2. Patients on linezolid may experience severe hypertension if large amounts of food containing tyramine are ingested.

_____ 3. Meropenem is contraindicated in patients allergic to cephalosporins and penicillins.

_____ 4. Flagyl works by lysing the cell wall of susceptible organisms.

_____ 5. Use of NebuPent may result in a metallic taste in the mouth.

_____ 6. Patients taking metronidazole should avoid alcoholic beverages during and for at least 1 day after treatment.

IV. MULTIPLE CHOICE

Circle the letter of the best answer.

1. Chloramphenicol works by ____.
   a. interfering with or inhibiting protein synthesis
   b. causing cell wall lysis
   c. overstimulating cell growth causing death of the microorganism
   d. depleting cellular glycogen stores
   e. None of the Above

2. Meropenem is used to treat ____.
   a. intra-abdominal infections
   b. bacterial meningitis
   c. pseudomembranous colitis
   d. oculitis
   e. Both a and b

3. The most serious adverse reactions of metronidazole involve the ____.
   a. gastrointestinal tract
   b. central nervous system
   c. ears
   d. kidneys
   e. liver

4. Pentamidine isethionate is used in the treatment of ____.
   a. *Enterobacter citrate*
   b. *Pseudomonas aeruginosa*
   c. *Pneumocystis jiroveci*
   d. methicillin-resistant *Staphylococcus aureus* (MRSA)
   e. amebiasis

5. Which miscellaneous anti-infective is only given by the intravenous route?
   a. Chloramphenicol
   b. Meropenem
   c. Linezolid
   d. Metronidazole
   e. Pentamidine isethionate

6. ____ may be given by aerosol.
   a. Chloramphenicol
   b. Meropenem
   c. Linezolid
   d. Metronidazole
   e. Pentamidine isethionate

7. Patients with gynecologic infections, such as trichomoniasis, may be treated with ____.
   a. chloramphenicol
   b. meropenem
   c. linezolid
   d. metronidazole
   e. pentamidine isethionate

V. RECALL FACTS

Indicate which of the following statements are facts with an F. If the statement is not a fact, leave the line blank.

ABOUT MISCELLANEOUS ANTI-INFECTIVES

____ 1. Meropenem is used to treat complicated skin and skin structure infections.

____ 2. Chloramphenicol interferes with or inhibits protein synthesis.

____ 3. Metronidazole is used to treat nosocomial pneumonia.

____ 4. Nephrotoxicity or ototoxicity may occur with vancomycin.

____ 5. Linezolid may be used in those with phenylketonuria.

____ 6. Phenobarbital or rifampin may increase chloramphenicol blood levels.

VI. FILL IN THE BLANKS

Fill in the blanks using words from the list below.

blood dyscrasias	meropenem	linezolid	vancomycin
intravenous	positive	pseudomembranous colitis	pentamidine isoethionate
thrombocytopenia	metronidazole		

1. The chief adverse reaction seen with the use of chloramphenicol is _____.

2. _____ is contraindicated in patients with phenylketonuria (PKU).

3. _____ can cause an abscess or phlebitis at the injection site.

4. Vancomycin acts against susceptible gram-_____ bacteria.

5. "Red man" syndrome refers to a severe adverse reaction associated with intravenous use of _____.

6. _____ may be given as an aerosol.

7. The more serious adverse reactions of linezolid are _____ and _____.

8. Meropenem is only given by the _____ route.

9. _____ may cause an unpleasant metallic taste.

VII. LIST

List the requested number of items.

1. List four uses of linezolid.

   a. _____

   b. _____

   c. _____

   d. _____

2. List six miscellaneous anti-infectives.

   a. _____

   b. _____

   c. _____

   d. _____

   e. _____

   f. _____

3. List six microorganisms that meropenem can be used to treat.

   a. _____

   b. _____

   c. _____

   d. _____

   e. _____

   f. _____

4. List five foods containing tyramine that should be avoided when taking linezolid.

   a. _____

   b. _____

   c. _____

   d. _____

   e. _____

VIII. CLINICAL APPLICATIONS

1. Mrs. P, a 75-year-old retired school teacher, has been prescribed an anti-infective drug to take when she leaves the hospital. What are key points about miscellaneous anti-infective drugs that she and her family members should know about?

IX. CASE STUDY

Mr. J. is being given intravenous vancomycin for his endocarditis. The health care team is monitoring him closely for any adverse reactions to this drug.

1. Which of the following are monitored closely while he is taking this drug?

   a. Infusion rate
   b. Blood pressure
   c. Fluid intake
   d. Output
   e. All of the above

2. Adverse reactions to vancomycin include all of the following except _____.

   a. elevated serum creatinine
   b. ototoxicity
   c. reversible neutropenia
   d. diarrhea

3. Mr. J. has begun to complain about throbbing neck pain. You think he may be experiencing red man syndrome. What other signs and symptoms may be associated with this?

   a. Decreased blood pressure
   b. Back pain
   c. Fever
   d. Chills
   e. Erythema of the neck and back
   f. All of the above

DRUGS THAT AFFECT THE IMMUNE SYSTEM

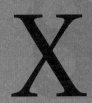

X

40

Immunological Agents

I. MATCH THE FOLLOWING

Match the term from Column A with the correct definition from Column B.

COLUMN A

___ 1. Antibody

___ 2. Antigen

___ 3. Attenuated

___ 4. Globulin

___ 5. Toxin

___ 6. Toxoid

___ 7. Vaccine

___ 8. Booster

COLUMN B

A. The administration of an additional dose of the vaccine to "boost" the production of antibodies to a level that will maintain the desired immunity

B. A poisonous substance produced by some bacteria

C. A toxin that is weakened but still capable of stimulating the formation of antitoxins

D. A substance, usually a protein, that stimulates the body to produce antibodies

E. Proteins present in blood serum or plasma that contain antibodies

F. A globulin produced by the B lymphocytes as a defense against an antigen

G. Weakened, as in the antigen strain used for vaccine development

H. Artificial active immunity created with killed or weakened antigens for the purpose of creating resistance to disease.

II. MATCH THE FOLLOWING

Match the term from Column A with the correct definition from Column B.

COLUMN A

_____ 1. Active immunity
_____ 2. Cell-Mediated immunity
_____ 3. Humoral immunity
_____ 4. Immunity
_____ 5. Passive immunity
_____ 6. Immune globulin

COLUMN B

A. Based on the antigen–antibody response, special lymphocytes produce circulating antibodies to act against a foreign substance.

B. The ability of the body to identify and resist micro-organism that are potentially harmful

C. The reaction of the body, when exposed to certain infectious microorganisms, of forming antibodies to the invading microorganism

D. Solutions obtained from human blood containing antibodies that have been formed by the body to specific antigen

E. A type of immunity occurring from the administration of ready-made antibodies from another individual or animal

F. The process of T lymphocytes and macrophages working together to destroy an antigen

III. MATCH THE FOLLOWING

Match the generic bacterial vaccine for active immunity from Column A with the correct trade name from Column B.

COLUMN A

_____ 1. Typhoid vaccine
_____ 2. Pneumococcal 7-valent conjugate vaccine
_____ 3. *Haemophilus influenza* type b conjugate and hepatitis B vaccine
_____ 4. Anthrax vaccine
_____ 5. Pneumococcal vaccine, polyvalent
_____ 6. *Haemophilus B* conjugate vaccine
_____ 7. Meningococcal polysaccharide vaccine

COLUMN B

A. Comvax
B. Biothrax
C. Act HIB
D. Prevnar
E. Pneumovax 23
F. Typhim VI
G. Menomune

IV. MATCH THE FOLLOWING

Match the generic viral vaccine from Column A with the correct trade name from Column B.

COLUMN A

_____ 1. Measles, mumps, and rubella virus vaccine, live

_____ 2. Human papillomavirus

_____ 3. Polio vaccine, inactivated

_____ 4. Hepatitis A, inactivated, and hepatitis B, recombinant vaccine

_____ 5. Rabies vaccine

_____ 6. Japanese encephalitis virus vaccine

_____ 7. Rotavirus vaccine

_____ 8. Varicella virus vaccine

_____ 9. Hepatitis B vaccine, recombinant

_____ 10. Hepatitis A vaccine

_____ 11. Zoster vaccine, live, attenuated

_____ 12. Influenza type A and B vaccine

COLUMN B

A. Zostavax

B. Rotarix

C. Afluria

D. IPOL

E. JE-Vax

F. MMR II

G. Havrix

H. Varivax

I. Twinrix

J. Engerix-B

K. Cervarix

L. Imovax

V. MATCH THE FOLLOWING

Match the generic immune globulin for passive immunity from Column A with the correct trade name from Column B.

COLUMN A

_____ 1. Rabies immune globulin, human

_____ 2. Cytomegalovirus immune globulin IV, human

_____ 3. Rh (D) immune globulin IV (human)

_____ 4. Antithymocyte globulin (rabbit)

_____ 5. Lymphocyte immune globulin, antithymocyte globulin (equine)

_____ 6. Immune globulin (human)

_____ 7. Botulism immune globulin IV

_____ 8. Hepatitis B immune globulin (human)

_____ 9. Immune globulin (human) subcutaneous

COLUMN B

A. Thymoglobulin

B. HyperRHO S/D

C. Hizentra

D. Atgam

E. BabyBIG

F. CytoGam

G. HepaGam B

H. GamaSTAN S/D

I. HyperRAB S/D

VI. MATCH THE FOLLOWING

Match the trade name from Column A with the type of immunity from Column B. You may use an answer more than once.

COLUMN A

_____ 1. Typhim VI
_____ 2. GamaSTAN S/D
_____ 3. Comvax
_____ 4. Act HIB
_____ 5. Atgam
_____ 6. Hizentra
_____ 7. HepaGam B
_____ 8. Menactra
_____ 9. HyperRAB
_____ 10. Carimune
_____ 11. CytoGam
_____ 12. BioThrax

COLUMN B

A. Active
B. Passive

VII. MATCH THE FOLLOWING

Match the trade name from Column A with the type of agent from Column B. You may use an answer more than once.

COLUMN A

_____ 1. BioThrax
_____ 2. WinRho SDF
_____ 3. Twinrix
_____ 4. Typhim VI
_____ 5. Kinrix
_____ 6. Atgam
_____ 7. CroFab
_____ 8. Pentacel
_____ 9. Comvax
_____ 10. CytoGam
_____ 11. YF-Vax
_____ 12. Zostavax
_____ 13. Vaqta
_____ 14. Decavac
_____ 15. Pediarix

COLUMN B

A. Bacterial vaccine
B. Viral vaccine
C. Toxoid
D. Immune globulin
E. Antivenin

VIII. TRUE OR FALSE

Indicate whether each statement is True (T) or False (F).

_____ 1. Active immunity involves agents that stimulate antibody formation.

_____ 2. Immunity is the resistance that an individual has against disease.

_____ 3. A vaccine that contains an attenuated antigen is one in which the antigen has been killed.

_____ 4. Many antigens, when killed, cause a good antibody response.

_____ 5. All forms of active immunity require booster shots.

_____ 6. Antibody-producing tissues cannot distinguish between a live or dead antigen.

_____ 7. Vaccines that contain weakened antigens are capable of causing disease in healthy individuals.

_____ 8. Vaccinations always result in a protective antibody response.

_____ 9. The administration of immune globulins is an example of passive immunity.

_____ 10. Adverse reactions of vaccines and toxoids are usually mild and subside within 48 hours.

_____ 11. The risk of serious adverse reactions from immunizations is much larger than the risk of contracting the same disease.

_____ 12. Immune globulins stimulate antibody production.

_____ 13. For the most effective response, antivenins should be administered within 4 hours after exposure.

_____ 14. A patient with isolated immunoglobulin A deficiency should not be given immune globulin preparations.

_____ 15. Antivenins are contraindicated in patients with hypersensitivity to horse serum or any component of the serum.

_____ 16. Antivenins have multiple known interactions.

_____ 17. All vaccines can be administered to those with minor illness, including a viral cold or a low-grade fever.

_____ 18. A postponement of the regular immunization schedule for children is never indicated.

_____ 19. After injection of immunizations, it is not uncommon to feel a lump at the injection site.

_____ 20. Only incidents that are positively related to an immunization should be reported to the Vaccine Adverse Event Reporting System (VAERS).

_____ 21. Immunizations required for travel should be given well in advance of departure so that adequate immunity is produced.

_____ 22. Serious viral infections of the CNS and fatalities have occurred with the use of some vaccines.

IX. MULTIPLE CHOICE

Circle the letter of the best answer.

1. _____ immunity occurs when a person is exposed to a disease, experiences the disease, and the body manufactures antibodies.
   a. Artificially acquired active
   b. Attenuated
   c. Passive
   d. Naturally acquired active
   e. Toxoid

2. Passive immunity _____.
   a. is obtained from the administration of immune globulins or antivenins
   b. provides immediate immunity
   c. lasts for a short time
   d. provides ready-made antibodies from another human or animal
   e. All of the above

3. Immunological agents may include _____.
   a. immune globulins
   b. toxoids

   c. vaccines
   d. Both a and b
   e. All of the above

4. A toxin is _____.
   a. capable of stimulating the body to produce antibodies
   b. capable of stimulating the body to produce antitoxins
   c. only able to stimulate the production of toxoids
   d. a way to produce antigens
   e. None of the Above

5. Vaccines and toxoids _____.
   a. are administered to stimulate the immune response in the body
   b. must be administered before exposure to the pathogenic organism
   c. provide passive immunity
   d. Both a and b
   e. Both a and c

6. Mr. C was given hepatitis B immune globulin 60 days ago after being exposed to the virus. He came into the office today to get an Engerix-B vaccine. What should the health care provider tell Mr. C?

   a. It is okay to get this vaccine today.
   b. Come back in another 30 days.
   c. The globulin preparation may interfere with your response to the vaccination.
   d. Both b and c
   e. Mr. C should never get this vaccine.

7. Insufficient antibodies may be produced when the immune system of a patient is depressed because of all but which of the following causes?

   a. Corticosteroids
   b. Salicylates
   c. Antineoplastic drugs
   d. Radiation therapy

8. Immune globulins _____.

   a. provide passive immunity to one or more infectious diseases
   b. produce a rapid onset of protection
   c. provide protection of short duration
   d. are generally given after exposure to the disease
   e. All of the above

9. Live virus vaccines should be administered 14 to 30 days before or _____.

   a. 6 to 12 weeks after administration of immunoglobulins
   b. 1 to 2 days after administration of immunoglobulins

   c. 8 to 10 months after administration of immunoglobulins
   d. not at all after administration of immunoglobulins
   e. 1 to 2 years after administration of immunoglobulins

10. After administration of an immunological agent, _____.

    a. a patient must be hospitalized for several days
    b. a patient may immediately go home
    c. a patient may be asked to remain on site for approximately 30 minutes
    d. a patient should eat a heavy fat meal
    e. None of the Above

11. _____ is (are) sometimes prescribed to control minor adverse reactions.

    a. Salicylates
    b. Narcotic agents
    c. Analeptics
    d. Acetaminophen
    e. Sedatives

12. The Vaccine Adverse Event Reporting System is a _____.

    a. local agency that monitors use of vaccines
    b. way to report health care provider carelessness
    c. national vaccine safety surveillance program
    d. program cosponsored by the CDC and the FDA
    e. Both c and d

X. RECALL FACTS

Indicate which of the following statements are facts with an F. If the statement is not a fact, leave the line blank.

ABOUT CONTRAINDICATIONS WITH THE MMR VACCINE

_____ 1. Lactation
_____ 2. First trimester of pregnancy
_____ 3. Allergic to neomycin
_____ 4. Allergic to gelatin
_____ 5. Corticosteroid therapy
_____ 6. Second or third trimester of pregnancy
_____ 7. Allergic reaction to previous dose of one of vaccines
_____ 8. Hypersensitive to an agent or components
_____ 9. Salicylate administration
_____ 10. Allergies to animals

ABOUT ADVERSE REACTIONS OF ANTIVENINS

_____ 1. Apprehension
_____ 2. Tingling fingers
_____ 3. Usually occur within 30 minutes of administration
_____ 4. Diarrhea
_____ 5. Cyanosis
_____ 6. Collapse
_____ 7. Clubbed fingers
_____ 8. Flushing
_____ 9. Itching and hives
_____ 10. Edema of the face, tongue, and throat

XI. FILL IN THE BLANKS

Fill in the blanks using words from the list below.

vaccines   increased   toxin   artificially acquired
passive   active   booster   globulins
antivenins   measles   mumps   rubella

1. _____ immunity involves the injection of ready-made antibodies found in the serum of immune individuals or animals.

2. _____ active immunity occurs when an individual is given a killed or weakened antigen that stimulates the formation of antibodies.

3. _____ injections help keep an adequate antibody titer circulating in the body.

4. _____ can contain either an attenuated or a killed antigen.

5. A _____ is a poisonous substance produced by some bacteria.

6. _____ immunity can be produced by administering vaccines or toxoids.

7. There is a(n) _____ risk of Reye syndrome when salicylates are administered with the varicella vaccine.

8. _____ are proteins present in blood serum or plasma that contain antibodies.

9. _____ are used for passive, transient protection from the toxic effects of bites by spiders and snakes.

10. Antibodies in immune globulin preparations may interfere with the immune response to live viral vaccines such as _____, _____, and _____.

XII. LIST

List the requested number of items.

1. List eight diseases for which there are vaccines available.

    a. _____

    b. _____

    c. _____

    d. _____

    e. _____

    f. _____

    g. _____

    h. _____

2. List five uses of vaccines and toxoids.

    a. _____

    b. _____

    c. _____

    d. _____

    e. _____

3. List five conditions in which vaccine and toxoid use are contraindicated.

    a. _____

    b. _____

    c. _____

    d. _____

    e. _____

4. List four types of bites for which antivenins are available.

    a. _____

    b. _____

    c. _____

    d. _____

5. List four types of patients who should not be given human immune globulin intravenous products.

    a. _____

    b. _____

    c. _____

    d. _____

XIII. CLINICAL APPLICATIONS

1. Mrs. C has been exposed to the hepatitis B virus by her husband and has been given Nabi-HB.

Explain to Mrs. C the most common adverse reactions of immune globulin therapy.

XIV. CASE STUDY

Ms. K. has brought her infant to the health care provider's office to receive routine immunizations. This is the first immunization the baby has received and

Ms. K. is asking many questions. You are trying to be thorough and cover all important aspects related to immunization.

1. You tell Ms. K. that the risks of contracting vaccine preventable diseases is _____ than the adverse reactions associated with immunizations.
   a. much higher
   b. much lower
   c. no different
   d. None of the above

2. You tell her that the following adverse reactions are common:
   a. Fever
   b. Nausea
   c. Vomiting
   d. Soreness at the injection site
   e. Both a and d

3. Treatment of these adverse reactions includes _____.
   a. narcotic administration
   b. acetaminophen
   c. warm compresses
   d. Both b and c
   e. None of the Above

41

Antineoplastic Drugs

I. MATCH THE FOLLOWING

Match the term from Column A with the correct definition from Column B.

COLUMN A

____ 1. Alopecia

____ 2. Anemia

____ 3. Extravasation

____ 4. Leukopenia

____ 5. Stomatitis

____ 6. Thrombocytopenia

____ 7. Oral Mucositis

____ 8. Vesicant

COLUMN B

A. Decrease in red blood cells

B. Inflammation of the oral mucous membranes

C. A decrease in the white blood cells or leukocytes

D. Inflammation of the mouth

E. An adverse drug reaction resulting in tissue necrosis

F. Escape of fluid from a blood vessel into surrounding tissues

G. The loss of hair

H. A decrease in the thrombocytes; a symptom of bone marrow depression

II. MATCH THE FOLLOWING

Match the alkylating drug or antibiotic generic name from Column A with the correct trade name from Column B.

COLUMN A

____ 1. epirubicin

____ 2. doxorubicin HCl

____ 3. streptozocin

____ 4. melphalan

____ 5. lomustine

____ 6. ifosfamide

____ 7. chlorambucil

____ 8. bendamustine

____ 9. dactinomycin

____ 10. idarubicin HCl

____ 11. valrubicin

____ 12. busulfan

COLUMN B

A. Adriamycin

B. Idamycin

C. Treanda

D. Busulfex

E. Leukeran

F. Alkeran

G. Ifex

H. Ellence

I. Valstar

J. CeeNU

K. Cosmegen

L. Zanosar

III. MATCH THE FOLLOWING

Match the generic antimetabolite or mitotic inhibitor from Column A with the correct trade name from Column B.

COLUMN A

	COLUMN B
____ 1. paclitaxel	A. Gemzar
____ 2. cladribine	B. Xeloda
____ 3. cytarabine	C. Nipent
____ 4. vincristine	D. DepoCyt
____ 5. pentostatin	E. Vincasar
____ 6. fludarabine	F. Fludara
____ 7. capecitabine	G. Leustatin
____ 8. docetaxel	H. Purinethol
____ 9. mercaptopurine	I. Taxotere
____ 10. gemcitabine HCl	J. Abraxane

IV. MATCH THE FOLLOWING

Match the generic androgen, antiandrogen, progestin, estrogen, antiestrogen, or gonadotropin-releasing hormone analogue from Column A with the correct trade name from Column B.

COLUMN A

	COLUMN B
____ 1. toremifene	A. Zytiga
____ 2. nilutamide	B. Fareston
____ 3. goserelin	C. Zoladex
____ 4. abiraterone acetate	D. Casodex
____ 5. fulvestrant	E. Faslodex
____ 6. leuprolide	F. Emcyt
____ 7. bicalutamide	G. Lupron
____ 8. triptorelin pamoate	H. Trelstar Depot
____ 9. estramustine	I. Depo-Provera
____ 10. medroxyprogesterone	J. Nilandron

V. MATCH THE FOLLOWING

Match the generic aromatase inhibitor, epipodophyllotoxin, enzyme, platinum coordination complex, anthracenedione, methylhydrazine derivative, or substituted urea from Column A with the correct trade name from Column B.

COLUMN A

	COLUMN B
____ 1. teniposide (VM-26)	A. Elspar
____ 2. procarbazine HCl	B. Femara
____ 3. letrozole	C. Eloxatin
____ 4. etoposide	D. Novantrone
____ 5. asparaginase	E. Droxia
____ 6. pegaspargase	F. Matulane
____ 7. hydroxyurea	G. Arimidex
____ 8. oxaliplatin	H. Vumon
____ 9. mitoxantrone	I. Toposar
____ 10. anastrazole	J. Oncaspar

VI. MATCH THE FOLLOWING

Match the generic cytoprotective agent, DNA topoisomerase inhibitor, biological response modifier, retinoid, or rexinoid from Column A with the correct trade name from Column B.

COLUMN A	COLUMN B
____ 1. irinotecan	A. Targretin
____ 2. bexarotene	B. Proleukin
____ 3. dexrazoxane	C. Hycamtin
____ 4. topotecan	D. Ontak
____ 5. aldesleukin	E. Zinecard
____ 6. amifostine	F. Ethyol
____ 7. tretinoin	G. Vesanoid
____ 8. levoleucovorin	H. Fusilev
____ 9. denileukin diftitox	I. TheraCys
____ 10. BCG, intravesical	J. Camptosar

VII. MATCH THE FOLLOWING

Match the generic monoclonal antibody or unclassified antineoplastic drug from Column A with the correct trade name from Column B.

COLUMN A	COLUMN B
____ 1. trastuzumab	A. Trisenox
____ 2. alemtuzumab	B. Herceptin
____ 3. ofatumumab	C. Lysodren
____ 4. mitotane	D. Photofrin
____ 5. arsenic trioxide	E. Arzerra
____ 6. ibritumomab tiuxetan	F. Zevalin
____ 7. porfimer sodium	G. Campath

VIII. MATCH THE FOLLOWING

Match the trade name from Column A with the drug type from Column B. You may use an answer more than once.

COLUMN A	COLUMN B
____ 1. Abraxane	A. Alkylating drug
____ 2. Xeloda	B. Antibiotic
____ 3. Matulane	C. Antimetabolite
____ 4. Hexalen	D. Mitotic inhibitor
____ 5. Ellence	E. Hormone
____ 6. Lupron	F. Miscellaneous anticancer drug
____ 7. Vumon	
____ 8. Leukeran	
____ 9. Clolar	
____ 10. Adriamycin	
____ 11. Targretin	
____ 12. Ifex	

IX. MATCH THE FOLLOWING

Match the drug form Column A with the use from Column B.

COLUMN A

_____ 1. Matulane
_____ 2. Leustatin
_____ 3. Eloxatin
_____ 4. Daunoxome
_____ 5. Photofrin
_____ 6. Myleran
_____ 7. CeeNU
_____ 8. Lysodren
_____ 9. Cosmegen

COLUMN B

A. Chronic myelogenous leukemia
B. Hairy cell leukemia
C. Hodgkin disease
D. Colon and colorectal cancer
E. Esophageal cancer
F. Adrenal cortical carcinoma
G. Brain tumors
H. Kaposi sarcoma
I. Wilms tumor

X. TRUE OR FALSE

Indicate whether each statement is True (T) or False (F).

_____ 1. Antineoplastic drugs always lead to a complete cure of the malignancy.

_____ 2. Chemotherapy refers to the use of antineoplastic drug therapy.

_____ 3. Antineoplastic drugs affect only the rapidly dividing cancer cells.

_____ 4. Alkylating drugs bind with DNA, causing breaks and thus preventing DNA replication.

_____ 5. Antineoplastic antibiotics have the same anti-infective ability as anti-infective antibiotics.

_____ 6. Methotrexate and fluorouracil are examples of antimetabolites.

_____ 7. Gonadotropin-releasing hormone analogues act by stimulating the anterior pituitary secretion of gonadotropins.

_____ 8. Single antineoplastic drugs often produce a better result than combination drug therapy.

_____ 9. An antiemetic can be given before administering an antineoplastic drug to help prevent nausea and vomiting.

_____ 10. All patients respond the same to antineoplastic drugs.

_____ 11. Doxorubicin can cause severe hair loss.

_____ 12. A patient who is experiencing nausea and vomiting as an adverse reaction should avoid greasy or fatty foods as well as unpleasant sights, smells, and tastes.

_____ 13. Extravasation of antineoplastic drugs has little effect on surrounding soft tissue.

_____ 14. Patients who are unable to communicate the pain they feel with extravasation are at greater risk.

_____ 15. Live virus vaccines generally produce an enhanced antibody production response when administered with fluorouracil or certain antineoplastic antibiotics.

_____ 16. Food decreases the absorption of fluorouracil.

_____ 17. Vitamin preparations containing folic acid may decrease the effects of methotrexate.

_____ 18. Bicalutamide may decrease the effect of oral anticoagulants.

_____ 19. Goserelin is administered subcutaneously into the soft tissue of the abdomen in a pellet form.

_____ 20. Green tea contains polyphenols or flavonoids.

XI. MULTIPLE CHOICE

Circle the letter of the best answer.

1. In which of the following areas are cells rapidly dividing and therefore may be affected by antineoplastic drug therapy?

   a. Mouth
   b. Gastrointestinal tract
   c. Gonads
   d. Bone marrow
   e. All of the above

2. According to the cell kill theory, ____.

   a. the first course of chemotherapy should kill 50% of the cancer cells
   b. the first course of chemotherapy should kill 80% of the cancer cells
   c. the first course of chemotherapy should kill 90% of the cancer cells
   d. the first course of chemotherapy should kill 100% of the cancer cells
   e. only one mega dose of an antineoplastic drug is needed to kill most types of cancer cells

3. All of the following are examples of alkylating drugs except ____.

   a. bleomycin sulfate
   b. busulfan
   c. chlorambucil
   d. melphalan
   e. thiotepa

4. Antineoplastic antibiotics ____.

   a. overstimulate cell growth causing cell death
   b. delay or inhibit cell division
   c. change the metabolism of the cell
   d. interfere with DNA and RNA synthesis
   e. Both b and d

5. Antimetabolites work by ____.

   a. inactivating enzymes
   b. altering the structure of DNA
   c. changing the DNA's ability to replicate
   d. All of the above
   e. Both b and c

6. Cisplatin is an example of a(n) ____ drug.

   a. alkylating
   b. miscellaneous antineoplastic
   c. antimetabolite
   d. antineoplastic antibiotic
   e. antimitotic

7. Adverse reactions to antineoplastic drugs are ____.

   a. sometimes dose dependent
   b. caused by the effect the drug has on many cells of the body
   c. of a wide variety
   d. sometimes desirable
   e. All of the above

8. Hyperuricemia may occur with ____.

   a. melphalan
   b. mercaptopurine
   c. plicamycin
   d. All of the above
   e. Both a and b

9. All of the following drugs except one cause gradual hair loss. Identify the exception.

   a. vinblastine
   b. vincristine
   c. etoposide
   d. bleomycin
   e. methotrexate

10. Bone marrow suppression as an adverse reaction to antineoplastic drug therapy can cause ____.

    a. anemia
    b. thrombocytopenia
    c. leukopenia
    d. leukocytosis
    e. All of the above

11. All of the following are signs of extravasation except ____.

    a. swelling
    b. stinging, burning, or pain at the injection site
    c. easy bruising
    d. redness
    e. lack of blood return

12. When cisplatin is used concurrently with ____, there is an increased risk of ototoxicity.

    a. antigout drugs
    b. cyclophosphamide
    c. loop diuretics
    d. aminoglycosides
    e. Both c and d

13. Which of the following antineoplastic antibiotics can cause an increased risk of bleeding when administered with aspirin, warfarin, heparin, or NSAIDs?

    a. plicamycin
    b. bleomycin
    c. mitomycin
    d. dactinomycin
    e. mitoxantrone

XII. RECALL FACTS

Indicate which of the following statements are facts with an F. If the statement is not a fact, leave the line blank.

ABOUT ANOREXIA AS AN ADVERSE REACTION

____ 1. Is a rare adverse reaction

____ 2. Is common with antineoplastic drug therapy

____ 3. Three large meals are better tolerated.

____ 4. Small, frequent meals are better tolerated.

____ 5. Breakfast is often the best tolerated meal.

____ 6. Lunch is often the best tolerated meal.

____ 7. Nutritional supplements may be prescribed.

____ 8. Patients' body weight is monitored weekly.

____ 9. Patients' body weight is monitored monthly.

ABOUT PATIENTS IN WHOM ANTINEOPLASTIC DRUGS ARE CONTRAINDICATED

____ 1. Leukopenia or thrombocytopenia

____ 2. Polycythemia

____ 3. Serious infections

____ 4. Anemia

____ 5. Serious renal disease

____ 6. Obesity

____ 7. Pregnancy

____ 8. Those who work with children

ABOUT PREGNANCY CATEGORY X DRUGS

____ 1. Levamisole

____ 2. Goserelin

____ 3. Triptorelin

____ 4. Thioguanine

____ 5. Plicamycin

____ 6. Flutamide

____ 7. Bicalutamide

____ 8. Methotrexate

____ 9. Vinblastine

____ 10. Dactinomycin

____ 11. Diethylstilbestrol

XIII. FILL IN THE BLANKS

Fill in the blanks using words from the list below.

intravenous	fluorouracil	earlier	antigout	less
tamoxifen	additive	stomatitis	temporary	antineoplastic
antimetabolites	mitotic inhibitor	treatment plan	alopecia	alkylating
dividing	gonadotropin-releasing hormone analogues			

1. _____ drugs can be used to cure, to control, or to provide palliative therapy of malignant tumors.

2. Chemotherapy is administered at the time the cell population is _____ to optimize cell death.

3. _____ drugs interfere with the process of cell division of both normal and malignant cells.

4. _____ disrupt normal cell functions by interfering with cellular metabolic functions.

5. _____ are used in the treatment of advanced prostatic carcinomas.

6. Vincristine is an example of a(n) _____.

7. A(n) _____ for antineoplastic drug therapy can prevent, lessen, or treat most of the symptoms of a specific adverse reaction.

8. _____ (hair loss) may affect a patient's mental health.

9. Hair loss from antineoplastic drug therapy is _____.

10. _____ or oral mucositis may occur 5 to 7 days after chemotherapy and continue up to 10 days after therapy.

11. The _____ extravasation is detected, the _____ likely soft tissue damage will occur.

12. _____ is not compatible with diazepam, doxorubicin, or methotrexate.

13. Antimetabolite and alkylating agents may antagonize _____ drugs by increasing serum uric acid levels.

14. Estrogens decrease the effectiveness of _____.

15. _____ bone marrow depressive effects occur when a mitotic inhibitor drug is administered with another antineoplastic drug.

16. The most common and reliable route of drug delivery is the _____ route.

XIV. LIST

List the requested number of items.

1. List five antineoplastic antibiotics.

   a. _____

   b. _____

   c. _____

   d. _____

   e. _____

2. List six common adverse reactions of antineoplastic drugs.

   a. _____

   b. _____

   c. _____

   d. _____

   e. _____

   f. _____

3. List four symptoms that indicate thrombocytopenia.

   a. _____

   b. _____

   c. _____

   d. _____

4. List three examples of vesicant drugs.

   a. _____

   b. _____

   c. _____

5. List five things that a patient should be assessed for following the administration of an antineoplastic drug.

   a. _____

   b. _____

   c. _____

   d. _____

   e. _____

6. List three antineoplastic drugs that are administered orally.

   a. _____

   b. _____

   c. _____

7. List five beneficial effects of green tea.

   a. _____

   b. _____

   c. _____

   d. _____

   e. _____

XV. CLINICAL APPLICATIONS

1. Mr. Y was recently diagnosed with esophageal cancer. His health care provider has chosen porfimer sodium (Photofrin) as part of his anti- neoplastic drug therapy. What adverse reactions might Mr. Y experience while receiving this medication?

XVI. CASE STUDY

Mr. K., a 60-year-old retired state worker, has been diag- nosed with advanced prostate cancer. His physician has started a regimen of triptorelin pamoate to treat him. This medication is administered as an intramuscular injection.

1. What is the treatment regimen commonly seen with this drug?
   a. 3.75 mg IM once every 4 weeks and 11.25 mg IM once every 12 weeks
   b. 2 mg IM twice per week for 4 weeks and 4 mg IM weekly thereafter
   c. 5 mg IM weekly for 3 weeks and 10 mg IM every month thereafter
   d. None of the above

2. Mr. K. could expect any of the following adverse reactions to this drug except _____.
   a. headache
   b. acne
   c. impotence
   d. edema in the legs

3. Precautions that Mr. K. should be given related to his being on antineoplastic drugs included which of the following?
   a. Keep all your appointments for chemotherapy.
   b. Do not take any nonprescription drugs unless approved by your health care provider.
   c. Do not drink alcoholic beverages unless your health care provider approves.
   d. All of the above.

XI

42

Musculoskeletal System Drugs

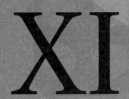

I. MATCH THE FOLLOWING

Match the term from Column A with the correct definition from Column B.

COLUMN A

____ 1. Chrysiasis

____ 2. Corticosteroids

____ 3. Gout

____ 4. Musculoskeletal

____ 5. Osteoarthritis

____ 6. Rheumatoid arthritis

COLUMN B

A. Gray to blue pigmentation of the skin that may occur from gold deposits in tissues.

B. A noninflammatory joint disease resulting in degeneration of the articular cartilage and changes in the synovial membrane

C. The bone and muscular structure of the body

D. A chronic disease characterized by inflammatory changes within the body's connective tissue

E. A form of arthritis in which uric acid accumulates in increased amounts in the blood and often is deposited in the joints

F. Hormones secreted from the adrenal cortex that contain potent anti-inflammatory action.

II. MATCH THE FOLLOWING

Match the generic drug name from Column A with the correct trade name from Column B.

COLUMN A

____ 1. allopurinol
____ 2. methocarbamol
____ 3. cyclobenzaprine hydrochloride
____ 4. leflunomide
____ 5. gold sodium, thiomalate
____ 6. zoledronic acid
____ 7. risedronate sodium
____ 8. alendronate sodium
____ 9. baclofen
____ 10. penicillamine
____ 11. metaxalone
____ 12. prednisone

COLUMN B

A. Myochrysine
B. Reclast
C. Flexeril
D. Intensol
E. Fosamax
F. Arava
G. Zyloprim
H. Cuprimine
I. Skelaxin
J. Actonel
K. Lioresal

III. MATCH THE FOLLOWING

Match the generic or trade name from Column A with the type of drug from Column B. You may use an answer more than once.

COLUMN A

____ 1. Enbrel
____ 2. Didronel
____ 3. Soma
____ 4. Azulfidine
____ 5. Zyloprim
____ 6. Dantrium
____ 7. Plaquenil sulfate
____ 8. Cuprimine
____ 9. colchicines
____ 10. Celestone
____ 11. Reclast
____ 12. Norflex

COLUMN B

A. Drugs used to treat osteoporosis
B. Drugs used to treat gout
C. Skeletal muscle relaxants
D. Corticosteroids
E. Miscellaneous drugs

IV. MATCH THE FOLLOWING

Match the generic drug name from Column A with the correct use from Column B. You may use an answer more than once.

COLUMN A

_____ 1. probenecid

_____ 2. dantrolene sodium

_____ 3. etidronate

_____ 4. prednisone

_____ 5. aurothioglucose

_____ 6. auranofin

_____ 7. orphenadrine citrate

_____ 8. baclofen

_____ 9. etanercept

_____ 10. sulfasalazine

_____ 11. tiludronate

_____ 12. leflunomide

COLUMN B

A. Paget disease

B. Rheumatoid arthritis

C. Gouty arthritis

D. Ankylosing spondylitis

E. Spasticity due to spinal cord injury

F. Discomfort due to musculoskeletal disorders

V. TRUE OR FALSE

Indicate whether each statement is True (T) or False (F).

_____ 1. Gold compounds suppress or prevent arthritis and synovitis.

_____ 2. Gold compounds can reverse structural changes to the joints.

_____ 3. A metallic taste may occur before stomatitis becomes evident when gold compounds are used.

_____ 4. Thrombocytopenia can occur with gold compound therapy.

_____ 5. Zyloprim acts by dissolving urate crystals in the joints.

_____ 6. Drugs used to treat gout are used to manage acute attacks or to prevent acute attacks.

_____ 7. Probenecid works by increasing the excretion of uric acid by the kidneys.

_____ 8. Patients being treated for gout should increase their fluid intake to approximately 3,000 ml/day.

_____ 9. Administration of allopurinol with aluminum salts may decrease the effectiveness of allopurinol.

_____ 10. Salicylates accelerate probenecid's uricosuric action.

_____ 11. There is a decreased incidence of skin rash when allopurinol and ampicillin are administered concurrently.

_____ 12. When a skeletal muscle relaxant is administered with alcohol, there is an increased CNS depressant effect.

_____ 13. Patients receiving hormone replacement therapy should not take bisphosphonates.

_____ 14. Alendronate bioavailability is increased when administered with ranitidine.

_____ 15. Absorption of bisphosphonates is increased when administered with calcium supplements or antacids.

_____ 16. Many adverse reactions are associated with high-dose and long-term corticosteroid therapy.

_____ 17. Any patient complaint related to penicillamine should be reported to the health care provider.

_____ 18. Any adverse reaction to hydroxychloroquine should immediately be reported to the health care provider.

_____ 19. Methotrexate is a Pregnancy Category X drug.

_____ 20. Patients who are allergic to penicillin can generally take penicillamine with no problems.

_____ 21. A total of 90% to 98% of the chondroitin molecules are absorbed.

_____ 22. Oral glucosamine theoretically provides a building block for regeneration of damaged cartilage.

_____ 23. No adverse reactions have been reported with glucosamine use.

_____ 24. Glucosamine and chondroitin are used to treat osteoarthritis.

_____ 25. Chondroitin molecules are large and therefore easily absorbed.

VI. MULTIPLE CHOICE

Circle the letter of the best answer.

1. Gold compound's ____.
   a. effects occur slowly
   b. mechanism of action is unknown
   c. adverse reactions may occur many months after therapy has been discontinued
   d. All of the above
   e. Both a and c

2. Chrysiasis ____.
   a. is caused by gold deposits in tissues
   b. is a reaction that causes gold crystal to form in the joints
   c. is the result of too large of a dose of a gold compound
   d. only occurs with auranofin
   e. is a gold pigmentation of the sclera

3. Which of the following treatments for gout works by reducing the production of uric acid?
   a. colchicine
   b. allopurinol
   c. sulfinpyrazone
   d. probenecid
   e. aurothioglucose

4. Which of the following drugs for gout is contraindicated in patients with peptic ulcer disease?
   a. gold compounds
   b. colchicines
   c. allopurinol
   d. sulfinpyrazone
   e. probenecid

5. ____ has an effect on muscle tone; therefore, it reduces muscle spasms.
   a. Soma
   b. Lioresal
   c. Flexeril
   d. Paraflex
   e. Valium

6. The most common adverse reaction of skeletal muscle relaxants is ____.
   a. gastrointestinal distress
   b. drowsiness
   c. skin rash
   d. ototoxicity
   e. hepatitis

7. The skeletal muscle relaxant that is contraindicated in patients with a recent myocardial infarction is ____.
   a. baclofen
   b. carisoprodol
   c. cyclobenzaprine
   d. dantrolene
   e. meprobamate

8. Which of the following bisphosphonate acts by inhibiting normal and abnormal bone resorption?
   a. alendronate
   b. etidronate
   c. risedronate
   d. All of the above
   e. Both b and c

9. ____ is used for postoperative treatment after total hip replacement.
   a. alendronate
   b. etidronate
   c. risedronate
   d. All of the above
   e. Both b and c

10. The mechanism of action of ____ is unknown in the treatment of rheumatoid arthritis.
    a. penicillamine
    b. methotrexate
    c. hydroxychloroquine
    d. All of the above
    e. Both a and c

11. Which of the following drugs are used to treat rheumatoid arthritis in patients who have had an insufficient therapeutic response to other antirheumatic drugs?
    a. penicillamine
    b. methotrexate
    c. hydroxychloroquine
    d. All of the above
    e. Both a and c

12. The drug ____ may have adverse effects on the eye as well as hematological effects.
    a. penicillamine
    b. methotrexate
    c. hydroxychloroquine
    d. allopurinol
    e. baclofen

13. The drug____ may cause an increase in skin friability.
    a. penicillamine
    b. methotrexate
    c. hydroxychloroquine
    d. allopurinol
    e. baclofen

14. The drug____ may cause abnormal hematology, liver function, or kidney function.
    a. penicillamine
    b. methotrexate
    c. hydroxychloroquine
    d. allopurinol
    e. baclofen

15. Therapy with musculoskeletal drugs may ____.
    a. keep the disorder under control
    b. improve the patient's daily living
    c. make the pain tolerable
    d. All of the above
    e. Both b and c

16. Glucosamine ____.
    a. is found in mucopolysaccharides, mucoproteins, and chitin
    b. is generally well tolerated
    c. is only used in combination with chondroitin
    d. All of the above
    e. Both a and b

VII. FILL IN THE BLANKS

Fill in the blanks using words from the list below.

decreases	skin rash	itching	unknown
bisphosphonates	hypocalcemia	90%–98%	methotrexate
Hyalgen	chondroitin	early	colchicine

1. The mechanism of action of gold compounds is _____.

2. The greatest benefit of gold compounds appears to occur in patients in the _____ stages of disease.

3. _____ may occur before a skin reaction to gold compounds and should be reported immediately.

4. Tolerance for gold therapy _____ with advancing age.

5. _____ has no effect on uric acid metabolism.

6. Allopurinol has been associated with _____ as an adverse reaction.

7. _____ are used to treat Paget disease.

8. Patients with _____ should not take alendronate or risedronate.

9. _____ is used to treat osteoarthritis knee pain and is administered directly into the knee.

10. _____ is used to treat severe disabling rheumatoid disease that is not responsive to other treatments.

11. _____ acts as the flexible connecting matrix between the protein filaments in cartilage.

12. Absorption of oral glucosamine is _____.

VIII. CLINICAL APPLICATIONS

1. Mrs. L has been prescribed a bisphosphonate for her postmenopausal osteoporosis. The health care provider has asked you to tell her how best to take this type of drug. Give Mrs. L some advice about taking this medication.

IX. CASE STUDY

Mr. N., age 35, was injured in a work-related construction accident. He has back and hip pain and is having difficulty walking. He is being prescribed a skeletal muscle relaxant, carisoprodol (Soma).

1. Mr. N. is asking you how this drug works. You would answer _____.
   a. the mode of action is not clearly understood
   b. the mode of action is inhibition of normal and abnormal bone resorption
   c. the mode of action is reduction of the production of uric acid
   d. None of the above

2. _____ is the most common reaction occurring with the use of skeletal muscle relaxants.
   a. Bone marrow depression
   b. Drowsiness
   c. Tachycardia
   d. Urate crystals in the joints

3. Mr. N. needs to be told key points about taking a skeletal muscle relaxant. These points include which of the following?
   a. Do not drive or perform other hazardous tasks if you feel drowsy.
   b. The drug is for short-term use.
   c. Do not use the drug for longer than 2 to 3 weeks.
   d. Avoid alcohol or other depressants while taking this drug.
   e. All of the above

43

Integumentary System Topical Drugs

I. MATCH THE FOLLOWING

Match the term from Column A with the correct definition from Column B.

COLUMN A

_____ 1. Antipsoriatics

_____ 2. Antiseptic

_____ 3. Bactericidal

_____ 4. Bacteriostatic

_____ 5. Keratolytic

_____ 6. Necrotic

_____ 7. Proteolysis

_____ 8. Purulent exudates

_____ 9. Superinfection

COLUMN B

A. A drug that stops, slows, or prevents the growth of microorganisms

B. A substance that destroys bacteria

C. A drug that removes excess growth of the epidermis in disorders such as warts

D. Drugs used to treat psoriasis

E. Dead, as in dead tissue

F. The slowing or retarding of the multiplication of bacteria

G. An overgrowth of bacterial or fungal microorganisms not affected by the antibiotic being administered

H. The process of hastening the reduction of proteins into simpler substances

I. Pus-containing fluid

II. MATCH THE FOLLOWING

Match the generic antibiotic or antipsoriatic drug name from Column A with the correct trade name from Column B.

COLUMN A

_____ 1. erythromycin

_____ 2. selenium sulfide

_____ 3. azelaic acid

_____ 4. metronidazole

_____ 5. sulfacetamide sodium

_____ 6. clindamycin

_____ 7. anthralin

_____ 8. calcipotriene

_____ 9. mupirocin

COLUMN B

A. Mexar

B. Psoriatec

C. Dandrex

D. Erymax

E. Cleocin T

F. Azelex

G. Bactroban

H. Dovonex

I. MetroLotion

III. MATCH THE FOLLOWING

Match the generic antifungal or antiviral drug from Column A with the trade name from Column B.

COLUMN A

_____ 1. docosanol
_____ 2. penciclovir
_____ 3. oxiconazole
_____ 4. butenafine
_____ 5. acyclovir
_____ 6. terbinafine
_____ 7. sulconazole
_____ 8. ketoconazole
_____ 9. sertaconazole
_____ 10. ciclopirox
_____ 11. naftifine
_____ 12. clotrimazole

COLUMN B

A. Zovirax
B. Mentax
C. Oxistat
D. Denavir
E. Ertaczo
F. Loprox
G. Nizoral
H. Lamisil
I. Exelderm
J. Naftin
K. Cruex
L. Abreva

IV. MATCH THE FOLLOWING

Match the generic antiseptic/germicide, enzyme preparation, keratolytic, or local anesthetic drug from Column A with the correct trade name from Column B.

COLUMN A

_____ 1. hexachlorophene
_____ 2. sodium hypochlorite
_____ 3. enzyme combination
_____ 4. povidone–iodine
_____ 5. pramoxine
_____ 6. chlorhexidine gluconate
_____ 7. masoprocol
_____ 8. collagenase
_____ 9. dibucaine
_____ 10. diclofenac

COLUMN B

A. Betadine
B. Santyl
C. Actinex
D. Hibiclens
E. Phiso-Hex
F. Dakin's solution
G. Solaraze
H. Nupercainal
I. Granulex
J. Caladryl

V. MATCH THE FOLLOWING

Match the generic topical corticosteroid from Column A with the correct trade name from Column B.

COLUMN A

_____ 1. augmented betamethasone dipropionate
_____ 2. desoximetasone
_____ 3. triamcinolone acetonide
_____ 4. fluocinolone acetonide
_____ 5. desonide
_____ 6. hydrocortisone butyrate
_____ 7. alclometasone dipropionate
_____ 8. mometasone furoate
_____ 9. hydrocortisone buteprate
_____ 10. flurandrenolide

COLUMN B

A. Diprolene
B. Capex
C. Locoid
D. Elocon
E. Kenalog
F. Pandel
G. Cordran
H. Aclovate
I. Desonate
J. Topicort

VI. MATCH THE FOLLOWING

Match the drug from Column A with the correct use from Column B.

COLUMN A

____ 1. Exelderm

____ 2. Granulex

____ 3. Metrolotion

____ 4. Nupercainal

____ 5. Azelex

____ 6. Taclonex

____ 7. Denavir

____ 8. Solaraze

____ 9. Bactroban

____ 10. Betasept

COLUMN B

A. Acne vulgaris

B. Rosacea

C. Impetigo

D. Tinea pedis, tinea cruris

E. Herpes labialis

F. Surgical scrub

G. Psoriasis

H. Actinic keratoses

I. Topical anesthesia

J. Debridement of necrotic tissue

VII. TRUE OR FALSE

Indicate whether each statement is True (T) or False (F).

____ 1. Topical anti-infectives include antibiotics, antifungals, and antiviral drugs.

____ 2. Topical antibiotics are only bacteriostatic.

____ 3. Antifungal drugs work by inhibiting the growth of fungi.

____ 4. Acyclovir is used as part of the initial treatment of genital warts.

____ 5. There are no significant interactions with the topical anti-infectives.

____ 6. An antiseptic works the same as a germicide.

____ 7. Except for econazole nitrate and ciclopirox, the pregnancy categories of the antifungals are unknown.

____ 8. Topical corticosteroids reduce itching, redness, and swelling when applied to inflamed skin.

____ 9. Topical antipsoriatics help remove the plaques associated with psoriasis.

____ 10. Numbness and dermatitis may occur as adverse reactions of topical enzymes.

____ 11. It is common practice to use topical enzymes to treat wounds in which nerves are exposed.

____ 12. Keratolytics are used to remove warts, calluses, corns, and seborrheic keratoses.

____ 13. Patients with diabetes or impaired circulation should not use keratolytics.

____ 14. Topical anesthetics may be applied to the skin or mucous membranes.

____ 15. Patients receiving Class I antiarrhythmic drugs should use tocainide cautiously.

____ 16. Adults older than 65 years generally have fewer skin-related adverse reactions to calcipotriene than younger adults.

____ 17. Aloe is used to prevent infection and promote healing of minor burns.

VIII. MULTIPLE CHOICE

Circle the letter of the best answer.

1. The drug ____ is used to treat eczema.

   a. Fungizone
   b. Caldecort
   c. penciclovir
   d. erythromycin
   e. Denavir

2. Which of the following is an example of a topical antibiotic?

   a. Micatin
   b. Zephiran
   c. Hibiclens
   d. Bacitracin
   e. Zovirax

3. The topical antiviral drugs currently available besides Zovirax include ____.

   a. penciclovir and docosanol
   b. hexachlorophene and amcinonide
   c. ciclopirox and fluocinomide
   d. amphotericin B and triamcinolone

4. Prolonged use of topical antibiotic preparations may result in a superficial ____.

   a. hypersensitivity reaction
   b. rash
   c. superinfection
   d. viral infection
   e. None of the above

5. ____ toxicity can cause ototoxicity and nephrotoxicity.

   a. acyclovir
   b. econazole nitrate
   c. penciclovir
   d. ciclopirox
   e. neomycin

6. Topical corticosteroids vary in potency because of the ____.

   a. concentration of the drug
   b. suspension vehicle
   c. area where the drug is applied
   d. All of the above
   e. Both a and c

7. Which of the following is not a topical corticosteroid?

   a. Aclovate
   b. Clobex
   c. Cordran
   d. Dandrex
   e. Pandel

8. Topical corticosteroids are contraindicated in which of the following situations?

   a. Known hypersensitivity
   b. As monotherapy for bacterial skin infections
   c. For use on the face, groin, or axilla
   d. For ophthalmic use
   e. All of the above

9. Topical anesthetics ____.

   a. may be applied to mucous membranes
   b. may be used to relieve itching and pain caused by skin conditions
   c. are commonly used for ophthalmic purposes
   d. All of the above
   e. Both a and b

10. A patient who is using lidocaine viscous should not eat food for 1 hour after use because ____.

   a. he or she may have impaired swallowing abilities and may aspirate
   b. the food will decrease the activity of the anesthetic
   c. the food will increase the absorption of the drug
   d. he or she will not be able to taste the food
   e. he or she may forget to chew

IX. RECALL FACTS

Indicate which of the following statements are facts with an F. If the statement is not a fact, leave the line blank.

ABOUT TOPICAL ANTISEPTICS AND GERMICIDES

____ 1. Chlorhexidine gluconate affects a wide range of microorganisms.

____ 2. Chlorhexidine gluconate can affect gram-negative and gram-positive bacteria.

____ 3. Benzalkonium solutions are bacteriostatic.

____ 4. Benzalkonium is active against bacteria, some viruses, fungi, and protozoa.

____ 5. Povidone–iodine is less preferred than iodine solution.

____ 6. Povidone–iodine–treated areas may be bandaged.

____ 7. Iodine is effective against many bacteria, fungi, viruses, yeasts, and protozoa.

____ 8. Topical antiseptics and germicides are only used on skin surfaces.

____ 9. Topical antiseptics and germicides have few adverse reactions.

____ 10. Topical antiseptics and germicides have no significant precautions or interactions when used as directed.

X. FILL IN THE BLANKS

Fill in the blanks using words from the list below.

hexachlorophene   synergistic   anthralin   C   aloe   keratolytics
B   topical enzymes   anti-inflammatory   bacteriostatic discontinuing

1. _____ drugs work by slowing or retarding the multiplication of bacteria.

2. Topical antibiotics are Pregnancy Category _____.

3. Topical corticosteroids exert localized _____ activity.

4. _____ may cause a temporary discoloration of the hair and fingernails.

5. _____ aid in the removal of dead soft tissue by hastening the reduction of proteins into smaller substances.

6. _____ may inhibit the activity of topical enzymes.

7. _____ are contraindicated for use on warts or mucous membranes.

8. Mexiletine and Class I antiarrhythmics have toxic effects that are potentially _____ when combined with topical anesthetics.

9. Adverse reactions caused by topical drugs can generally be relieved by _____ the drug.

10. _____ is an herb that helps repair skin tissue and reduce inflammation.

XI. LIST

List the requested number of items.

1. List three topical antifungal drugs used to treat tinea pedis, tinea cruris, tinea corporis, and superficial candidiasis.

   a. _____
   b. _____
   c. _____

2. List five adverse reactions to topical anti-infectives.

   a. _____
   b. _____
   c. _____
   d. _____
   e. _____

3. List five uses of topical corticosteroids.

   a. _____
   b. _____

   c. _____
   d. _____
   e. _____

4. List three conditions that may be treated with a topical enzyme.

   a. _____
   b. _____
   c. _____

5. List five uses of aloe.

   a. _____
   b. _____
   c. _____
   d. _____
   e. _____

XII. CLINICAL APPLICATIONS

1. Ms. G has been using a topical corticosteroid to help manage a skin condition. She has noted that the area seems to be dry and is itching more. What might Ms. G do to help relieve this adverse reaction to the medication?

XIII. CASE STUDY

Mr. S. has been taking a keratolytic medication to assist with the removal of seborrheic keratoses. He has come back to the office complaining of dry skin and experiencing excessive itching.

1. Which of the following interventions would help with this dry skin problem?

    a. Keep the nails short
    b. Use warm water with mild soap for cleaning the skin, and rinse and dry the skin thoroughly
    c. Bath oils, creams, and lotions may be applied if necessary as long as the health care provider is consulted first
    d. All of the above

2. The drug Mr. S. is taking is diclofenac sodium. All of the following are possible adverse reactions seen with this drug except _____.

    a. erythema
    b. rash
    c. dry skin
    d. flu syndrome

3. For his keratosis, the drug order would read _____.

    a. apply daily for 10 days.
    b. apply three times per day after meals
    c. apply at bedtime
    d. apply to affected area two times per day

44

Otic and Ophthalmic Preparations

I. MATCH THE FOLLOWING

Match the term from Column A with the correct definition from Column B.

COLUMN A

____ 1. Cycloplegia

____ 2. Miosis

____ 3. Miotic

____ 4. Mydriasis

____ 5. Mydriatics

____ 6. Otic

COLUMN B

A. Drugs that dilate the pupil, constrict superficial blood vessels of the sclera, and decrease the formation of aqueous humor

B. Dilation of the pupil

C. Paralysis of the ciliary muscle, resulting in an inability to focus the eye

D. Ear

E. Drugs used to help contract the pupil of the eye

F. The contraction of the pupil of the eye.

II. MATCH THE FOLLOWING

Match the trade name of the otic preparation from Column A with the type of preparation from Column B. You may use an answer more than once.

COLUMN A

____ 1. Aural

____ 2. Cortisporin Otic

____ 3. Derm Otic

____ 4. Cetraxal

____ 5. Acetasol HCL

____ 6. Cipro HC Otic

____ 7. Aero Otic

____ 8. Ciprodex

____ 9. Zinotic

____ 10. Pro-Otic

COLUMN B

A. Steroid and antibiotic combination solutions

B. Steroid and antibiotic combinations, suspensions

C. Otic antibiotics

D. Select miscellaneous preparations

III. MATCH THE FOLLOWING

Match the generic ophthalmic drug name from Column A with the correct trade name from Column B.

COLUMN A	COLUMN B
____ 1. betaxolol	A. Betoptic
____ 2. carbachol	B. Azopt
____ 3. travoprost	C. Isopto-Carbachol
____ 4. ketorolac tromethamine	D. Alamast
____ 5. scopolamine	E. Iopidine
____ 6. brinzolamide	F. Isopto Hyoscine
____ 7. pilocarpine	G. Ak-Dilate
____ 8. apraclonidine	H. Betimol
____ 9. loteprednol	I. Travatan Z
____ 10. pemirolast	J. Isopto-Carpine
____ 11. timolol	K. Alrex
____ 12. phenylephrine	L. Acular

IV. MATCH THE FOLLOWING

Match the generic ophthalmic drug name from Column A with the correct trade name from Column B.

COLUMN A	COLUMN B
____ 1. gentamicin	A. Natacyn
____ 2. dexamethasone	B. Trusopt
____ 3. natamycin	C. Maxidex
____ 4. dorzolamide	D. Flarex
____ 5. atropine sulfate	E. Isopto-Atropine
____ 6. prednisolone	F. Ilotycin
____ 7. brimonidine tartrate	G. Visine L.R.
____ 8. fluorometholone	H. Omnipred
____ 9. oxymetazoline hydrochloride	I. Alphagan
____ 10. erythromycin	J. Garamycin

V. MATCH THE FOLLOWING

Match the ophthalmic preparation trade name from Column A with the type of preparation from Column B.

COLUMN A

____ 1. Phospholine Iodide
____ 2. Tobrasol
____ 3. Isopto Carbachol
____ 4. Maxidex
____ 5. Trusopt
____ 6. Voltaren
____ 7. Betimol
____ 8. Zirgan
____ 9. Isopto Homatropine
____ 10. Alocril
____ 11. Alphagan
____ 12. Lumigan
____ 13. Cyclomydril
____ 14. Iopidine
____ 15. Natacyn

COLUMN B

A. Alpha 2-adrenergic agonist
B. Sympathomimetics
C. Cycloplegic/mydriatics
D. Beta-adrenergic blocking drugs
E. Miotics, direct acting
F. Miotics, cholinesterase inhibitors
G. Carbonic anhydrase inhibitors
H. Prostaglandin agonist
I. Mast cell stabilizer
J. NSAID
K. Corticosteroids
L. Antibiotics
M. Vasoconstrictors/mydriatics
N. Antiviral drugs
O. Antifungal drugs

VI. MATCH THE FOLLOWING

Match the ophthalmic preparation from Column A with the correct use from Column B.

COLUMN A

____ 1. Phospholine Iodide
____ 2. Ilotycin
____ 3. Alamast
____ 4. Betoptic
____ 5. Ocufen
____ 6. Natacyn
____ 7. Alphagen P
____ 8. Isopto–Carpine
____ 9. Viroptic
____ 10. Garamycin

COLUMN B

A. Treatment of fungal eye infections
B. Prevention of ophthalmia neonatorum
C. Treatment of eye infections
D. Allergic conjunctivitis
E. Glaucoma
F. Treatment of herpes simplex keratitis
G. Chronic open-angle glaucoma
H. Elevated IOP
I. Glaucoma and strabismus
J. Inhibition of intraoperative miosis

VII. TRUE OR FALSE

Indicate whether each statement is True (T) or False (F).

____ 1. Miscellaneous preparations for the treatment of otic conditions may contain antipyrine.

____ 2. Otic preparations are used to treat inner ear infections.

____ 3. It is safe to use drugs to remove cerumen at any time.

____ 4. No significant drug interactions have been reported with the use of otic preparations.

____ 5. The incidence of adverse reactions associated with ophthalmic drugs is usually small.

____ 6. Brimonidine tartrate is used to treat open-angle glaucoma or ocular hypertension.

_____ 7. Sympathomimetic drugs lower intraocular pressure by increasing the outflow of aqueous humor in the eye.

_____ 8. Systemic reactions never occur with sympathomimetic drugs used to treat ocular conditions.

_____ 9. When beta-adrenergic drugs for ophthalmic purposes are administered with oral beta-blockers, there may be an increased or additive effect of the drugs.

_____ 10. Cholinesterase inhibitors cause an increased resistance to aqueous flow.

_____ 11. Systemic toxicity (i.e., nausea, vomiting, diarrhea) occurs more often with cholinesterase inhibitors than with miotics.

_____ 12. Carbonic anhydrase inhibitors are used in the treatment of elevated intraocular pressure seen in open-angle glaucoma.

_____ 13. Carbonic anhydrase inhibitors are contraindicated during pregnancy and lactation.

_____ 14. Prostaglandin agonists are contraindicated during pregnancy.

_____ 15. Mast cell stabilizers work by stimulating the release of anti-inflammatory mediators.

_____ 16. Ketorolac is a nonsteroidal anti-inflammatory drug used for the relief of itching of eyes caused by seasonal allergies.

_____ 17. A patient who has had a superficial corneal foreign body should not be given a corticosteroidal ophthalmic preparation.

_____ 18. Antiviral drugs interfere with DNA synthesis.

_____ 19. Antifungal drugs can act against yeast.

_____ 20. Systemic adverse reactions of ophthalmic vasoconstrictors and mydriatics can include headaches, tachycardia, and stroke.

_____ 21. Cycloplegic mydriatics cause paralysis of the ciliary muscle.

_____ 22. Cycloplegic mydriatics have had no significant drug interactions reported when the drugs are given topically.

VIII. MULTIPLE CHOICE

Circle the letter of the best answer.

1. Carbamide peroxide found in miscellaneous otic preparations is used to _____.
   a. provide antifungal action
   b. provide analgesia
   c. prevent inflammation
   d. help remove ear wax
   e. produce local anesthesia

2. Ophthalmic preparations may be used for _____.
   a. lowering intraocular pressure
   b. bacterial or viral infections
   c. inflammatory conditions
   d. symptoms of allergy related to the eye
   e. All of the above

3. The drug _____ is an alpha 2-adrenergic receptor agonist.
   a. apraclonidine
   b. brimonidine
   c. epinephrine
   d. dipivefrin
   e. dapiprazole

4. Patients taking _____ should not use brimonidine tartrate.
   a. oral contraceptives
   b. estrogen replacement therapy
   c. monoamine oxidase inhibitors
   d. antibiotics
   e. oral anticoagulants

5. The drug _____ is used to control or prevent postoperative elevations in intraocular pressure.
   a. apraclonidine
   b. brimonidine tartrate
   c. dapiprazole
   d. dorzolamide
   e. ketorolac

6. Bepreve is used to _____.
   a. reverse diagnostic mydriasis
   b. block the beta-adrenergic receptors causing dilation of the iris
   c. inhibit narrow-angle glaucoma
   d. reduce the production of tears
   e. None of the above

7. In which of the following conditions are beta-adrenergic blocking drugs contraindicated?
   a. Acute iritis
   b. Pregnancy
   c. Sinus bradycardia
   d. Conjunctivitis
   e. Ptosis

8. Cholinesterase inhibitors are used to treat _____.
   a. open-angle glaucoma
   b. closed-angle glaucoma
   c. iritis
   d. conjunctivitis
   e. retinal detachment

9. Iris cysts may form in patients taking cholinesterase inhibitors but will usually shrink ____.
   a. after discontinuation of the drug
   b. after a reduction in frequency of instillation
   c. after a reduction in strength of the drops
   d. All of the above
   e. None of the above; iris cysts are permanent.

10. Prostaglandin agonists are used ____.
    a. to lower intraocular pressure
    b. to raise intraocular pressure
    c. to increase the flow of aqueous humor out of the eye
    d. Both a and b
    e. Both a and c

11. Mast cell stabilizers are used for ____.
    a. blurred vision correction
    b. the prevention of eye itching caused by allergic conjunctivitis
    c. lowering intraocular pressure
    d. treatment of macular degeneration
    e. treatment of night blindness

12. In which of the following patients is the use of a mast cell stabilizer contraindicated?
    a. A patient who wears colored contact lenses
    b. A patient with open-angle glaucoma
    c. A patient with a hypersensitivity to the medication
    d. All of the above
    e. Both a and c

13. Which of the following nonsteroidal anti-inflammatory drug might be chosen to prevent miosis during eye surgery?
    a. diclofenac
    b. ketorolac
    c. nedocromil
    d. flurbiprofen
    e. pemirolast

14. Nonsteroidal anti-inflammatory drugs used for ophthalmic purposes have as their most common adverse reaction ____.
    a. transient burning and stinging
    b. discoloration of contact lenses
    c. increased intraocular pressures
    d. iritis
    e. dry eyes

15. Which of the following are potential adverse reactions of corticosteroid use?
    a. Elevated intraocular pressure
    b. Loss of visual acuity
    c. Cataract formation
    d. Delayed wound healing
    e. All of the above

16. Vasoconstrictors and mydriatics can act to ____.
    a. dilate the pupil
    b. constrict superficial blood vessels of the sclera
    c. decrease the formation of aqueous humor
    d. All of the above
    e. Both a and b

17. A patient needing to have his or her pupils dilated for examination of the eye may be given a ____.
    a. sympathomimetic
    b. nonsteroidal anti-inflammatory drug
    c. corticosteroid
    d. mydriatic
    e. miotic

18. Vasoconstrictors and mydriatics would be contraindicated in a patient with ____.
    a. sulfite sensitivity
    b. iritis
    c. narrow-angle glaucoma
    d. Both a and c
    e. Both a and b

19. Cycloplegic mydriatics are used ____.
    a. to treat inflammatory conditions of the iris
    b. to treat inflammatory conditions of the uveal tract
    c. for examination of the eye
    d. All of the above
    e. None of the above

20. Inactive ingredients in artificial tears may include which of the following?
    a. Preservatives
    b. Antioxidants
    c. Drugs that slow drainage
    d. All of the above
    e. Both a and c

IX. RECALL FACTS

Indicate which of the following statements are facts with an F. If the statement is not a fact, leave the line blank.

ABOUT PATIENT MANAGEMENT ISSUES WITH OPHTHALMIC PREPARATIONS

_____ 1. Ophthalmic ointments are applied to the eyelids or dropped into the lower conjunctival sac.

_____ 2. Ophthalmic solutions are applied under the eyelid.

_____ 3. When applying two eye drop prescriptions at the same time, wait at least 5 minutes before instilling the second drug.

_____ 4. Ophthalmic drugs may produce blurred vision.

_____ 5. Any liquid medication can be applied to the eye.

_____ 6. Sympathomimetic ophthalmic drugs can cause systemic effects in patients.

_____ 7. Visual impairment caused by ophthalmic drugs never lasts more than 30 minutes.

_____ 8. Ophthalmic drug containers can be warmed in the hands before instilling the drug.

X. FILL IN THE BLANKS

Fill in the blanks using words from the list below.

miotics	adrenochrome	impaired	respiratory tract	prostaglandin
natamycin	mydriatics	artificial tear	systemically	nedocromil
pemirolast	diclofenac	corticosteroids	superinfection	reduced

1. Prolonged use of otic preparations containing an antibiotic may result in a(n) _____.

2. Patients using otic preparations should be told that hearing in the treated ear may be _____ while the solution remains in the ear canal.

3. Brimonidine tartrate works by _____ aqueous humor production.

4. Prolonged use of sympathomimetic drugs for treatment of ocular disorders may result in _____ deposits in the cornea and conjunctiva.

5. _____ contract the pupil of the eye.

6. Persons working with insecticides containing carbamate or organophosphate are at risk for systemic effects of cholinesterase inhibitors because of absorption through the _____ or the skin.

7. Most carbonic anhydrase inhibitors are administered _____.

8. Mast cell stabilizers currently used for ophthalmic use are _____ and _____.

9. _____ can be used to treat postoperative inflammation after eye surgery.

10. Nonsteroidal anti-inflammatory drugs work by inhibiting _____ synthesis.

11. Prolonged use of _____ may result in elevated intraocular pressure and nerve damage.

12. _____ is the only ophthalmic antifungal drug in use.

13. Exaggerated adrenergic effects may occur when _____ are administered with MAOIs.

14. _____ solutions lubricate the eyes and can be used to treat dry eyes.

XI. LIST

List the requested number of items.

1. List the three categories of otic preparations.

   a. _____

   b. _____

   c. _____

2. List four uses of otic preparations.

   a. _____

   b. _____

   c. _____

   d. _____

3. List four conditions in which drugs to remove cerumen should not be used.

   a. _____

   b. _____

   c. _____

   d. _____

4. List five transient local reactions to sympathomimetic drugs.

   a. _____

   b. _____

   c. _____

   d. _____

   e. _____

5. List five adverse reactions of carteolol.

   a. _____

   b. _____

   c. _____

   d. _____

   e. _____

6. List five conditions in which direct acting miotics are used with caution.

   a. _____

   b. _____

   c. _____

   d. _____

   e. _____

7. List five ophthalmic uses of corticosteroids.

   a. _____

   b. _____

   c. _____

   d. _____

   e. _____

8. List three uses of antiviral drugs in ophthalmic disorders.

   a. _____

   b. _____

   c. _____

9. List five systemic adverse reactions of cycloplegic mydriatics.

   a. _____

   b. _____

   c. _____

   d. _____

   e. _____

XII. CLINICAL APPLICATIONS

1. Mrs. P, age 76, has been to see her health care provider to be treated for decreased hearing. After determining that there is no infection at the site, her health care provider decides that her hearing loss is due to wax buildup. Using the summary drug table of otic preparations, choose a medication that will be effective and easy for her to instill by herself.

XIII. CASE STUDY

Mr. P., age 80, has come to his physician with a complaint of itching and redness of his left eye. Upon examination, his doctor has decided he has allergic conjunctivitis. The physician has ordered a corticosteroid medication, Maxidex ointment, to be used for this condition.

1. What is the mechanism of action that makes this drug effective for conjunctivitis?

    a. Mydriasis
    b. Anti-inflammatory activity
    c. Miosis
    d. Action against a variety of yeast and fungi

2. All of the following are adverse reactions to corticosteroid ophthalmic preparations except _____.

    a. elevated intraocular pressure
    b. loss of visual acuity
    c. nausea and vomiting
    d. foreign body sensation

3. Mr. P. is being instructed about application of the Maxidex ointment. Which of the following information would be included?

    a. Ointments are applied to the eyelids or dropped into the lower conjunctival sac.
    b. Temporary blurring of vision may occur.
    c. Do not rub your eyes, and keep your hands away from your eyes.
    d. All of the above.

45

Fluids, Electrolytes, and Total Parenteral Nutrition

I. MATCH THE FOLLOWING

Match the term from Column A with the correct definition from Column B.

COLUMN A

____ 1. Electrolyte

____ 2. Extravasation

____ 3. Half-normal saline

____ 4. Hypocalcemia

____ 5. Hypokalemia

____ 6. Hyponatremia

____ 7. Normal saline

____ 8. Protein substrates

COLUMN B

A. An electrically charged particle that is essential for normal cell function and is involved in various metabolic activities

B. Low blood calcium

C. Solution containing 0.45% NaCl

D. Solution containing 0.9% NaCl

E. Escape of fluid from a vessel into surrounding tissues

F. Amino acid preparations that act to promote the production of proteins and are essential to life

G. Low blood sodium

H. Low blood potassium

II. MATCH THE FOLLOWING

Match the electrolyte imbalance from Column A with the signs and symptoms from Column B.

COLUMN A

____ 1. Hypocalcemia

____ 2. Hypercalcemia

____ 3. Hypomagnesemia

____ 4. Hypermagnesemia

____ 5. Hypokalemia

____ 6. Hyperkalemia

____ 7. Hyponatremia

____ 8. Hypernatremia

COLUMN B

A. Anorexia, nausea, vomiting, ECG changes

B. Leg and foot cramps, hypertension, tachycardia

C. Lethargy, drowsiness, impaired respiration

D. Fever, hot-dry skin, dry, sticky mucous membranes

E. Hyperactive reflexes, muscle twitching, muscle cramps, tetany

F. Cold, clammy skin, decreased skin turgor, apprehension

G. Irritability, anxiety, listlessness, mental confusion

H. Anorexia, nausea, bone tenderness, polyuria, polydipsia, cardiac arrest

III. MATCH THE FOLLOWING

Match the information from Column A with the correct electrolyte from Column B. You may use an answer more than once.

COLUMN A

____ 1. Used in the treatment of metabolic acidosis

____ 2. Is important in the transmission of nerve impulses

____ 3. Used for blood clotting and bone and teeth building

____ 4. Contraction of smooth, cardiac, and skeletal muscles

____ 5. Used as a gastric and urinary alkalinizer

____ 6. May decrease the absorption of ketoconazole

____ 7. Used in the treatment of hypocalcemia

____ 8. Used to treat hypokalemia

____ 9. Maintenance of normal heart action

____ 10. Used in half-normal and normal saline

____ 11. Can cause local tissue necrosis if extravasation occurs

____ 12. Is contraindicated in patients with hypercalcemia, with ventricular fibrillation, or who are taking digitalis

COLUMN B

A. Bicarbonate

B. Calcium

C. Magnesium

D. Potassium

E. Sodium

IV. TRUE OR FALSE

Indicate whether each statement is True (T) or False (F).

____ 1. No interactions have been reported in the use of blood plasma.

____ 2. Plasma protein fractions are administered intramuscularly.

____ 3. A blood type and cross-match are not needed when plasma protein fractions are given.

____ 4. Protein substrates have no known adverse reactions.

____ 5. Energy substrates include dextrose solutions and fat emulsions.

____ 6. No more than 60% of a patient's total caloric intake should come from fat emulsion.

____ 7. Fat emulsions are used in patients requiring parenteral nutrition for extended periods.

____ 8. Plasma expanders can be used as a substitute for whole blood or plasma in the treatment of shock.

____ 9. Fat solution infusion patients should be carefully observed during the first 30 minutes of infusion for signs of a reaction.

____ 10. Periodic serum electrolyte levels should be used to monitor electrolyte therapy.

____ 11. Peripheral total parenteral nutrition is used in patients who are severely hypercatabolic.

____ 12. Hyperglycemia is the most common metabolic complication of total parenteral nutrition.

V. MULTIPLE CHOICE

Circle the letter of the best answer.

1. Human plasma is used to ____.
   a. replace red blood cell volume
   b. increase blood volume
   c. replace plasma proteins
   d. restore electrolyte balance
   e. protect against transfusion reactions

2. Serum albumin ____.
   a. is obtained from donated whole blood
   b. is a protein found in plasma
   c. can be artificially produced
   d. Both a and b
   e. Both b and c

3. Plasma protein fractions are used to treat ____.
   a. hypervolemic shock
   b. hypovolemic shock
   c. hypoproteinemia
   d. Both a and c
   e. Both b and c

4. Protein substrates ____.
   a. are amino acid preparations that act to promote the production of proteins
   b. are commonly given to treat kidney failure
   c. will cure congestive heart failure
   d. decrease the production of proteins by the body
   e. None of the above

5. Energy substrate solutions include ____.
   a. dextrose solutions
   b. fat emulsions
   c. blood plasma
   d. All of the above
   e. Both a and b

6. Dextrose solutions ____.
   a. are contraindicated in patients with diabetic coma and with high blood sugar levels
   b. are used cautiously in patients receiving a corticosteroid
   c. are incompatible with blood
   d. can be in a concentrated form
   e. All of the above

7. Hetastarch may cause ____.
   a. vomiting
   b. diarrhea
   c. blurred vision
   d. seizures
   e. ototoxicity

8. Plasma expanders are contraindicated in all of the following patients except those with ____.
   a. severe bleeding disorders
   b. severe cardiac failure
   c. Parkinson disease
   d. renal failure with oliguria
   e. renal failure with anuria

9. Intravenous replacement solutions ____.
   a. are a source of electrolytes
   b. are a source of water
   c. are used to facilitate amino acid utilization
   d. maintain electrolyte balance
   e. All of the above

10. Pedialyte ____.
    a. contains carbohydrates and electrolytes
    b. is an oral electrolyte solution
    c. is used to treat severe vomiting or diarrhea
    d. replaces lost electrolytes, carbohydrates, and fluids
    e. All of the above

11. Total parenteral nutrition is used to ____.
    a. prevent weight loss
    b. prevent nitrogen loss
    c. treat negative nitrogen balance
    d. All of the above
    e. Both b and c

12. A hyperglycemic reaction to total parenteral nutrition may be dealt with by ____.
    a. decreasing the rate of administration
    b. reducing the dextrose concentration
    c. administering insulin
    d. All of the above
    e. None of the above

VI. RECALL FACTS

Indicate which of the following statements are facts with an F. If the statement is not a fact, leave the line blank.

ABOUT PATIENT MANAGEMENT ISSUES WITH ELECTROLYTE THERAPY

_____ 1. Bicarbonate is used to treat respiratory acidosis.

_____ 2. Systemic overloading of calcium can cause weakness, lethargy, severe nausea and vomiting, and coma.

_____ 3. Potassium is irritating to tissues.

_____ 4. Patients receiving magnesium sulfate must be observed constantly.

_____ 5. Intravenous sodium chloride solutions can cause pulmonary edema.

_____ 6. Oral sodium bicarbonate should be taken with milk.

_____ 7. Oral potassium tablets should be chewed.

_____ 8. Direct intravenous injection of potassium can result in sudden death.

_____ 9. Magnesium sulfate can be given intramuscularly or intravenously.

_____ 10. Older adults should receive a standard dose of magnesium; only children receive a lower dose.

VII. FILL IN THE BLANKS

Fill in the blanks using words from the list below.

total parenteral nutrition   electrolytes   plasma expanders
fat emulsion   plasma protein fractions   fluid overload

1. _____ include human plasma protein fraction and normal serum albumin.

2. An intravenous _____ contains soybean or safflower oil and a mixture of natural triglycerides.

3. _____ are used to expand plasma volume.

4. A common adverse reaction to all solutions administered by the parenteral route is _____.

5. Some _____ may cause cardiac irregularities.

6. _____ may be administered through a peripheral vein or through a central venous catheter.

VIII. LIST

List the requested number of items.

1. List three functions of the albumin fraction of human blood.

   a. _____

   b. _____

   c. _____

2. List five conditions in which plasma proteins are contraindicated.

   a. _____

   b. _____

   c. _____

   d. _____

   e. _____

3. List the two most common adverse reactions associated with the administration of fat emulsions.

   a. _____

   b. _____

4. List three intravenous solutions of plasma expanders.

   a. _____

   b. _____

   c. _____

5. List four uses of calcium.

    a. _____

    b. _____

    c. _____

    d. _____

6. List five examples of combined intravenous electrolyte solutions.

    a. _____

    b. _____

    c. _____

    d. _____

    e. _____

7. List five products that can be used to meet the intravenous nutritional requirements of a patient.

    a. _____

    b. _____

    c. _____

    d. _____

    e. _____

8. List five symptoms of fluid overload.

    a. _____

    b. _____

    c. _____

    d. _____

    e. _____

9. List five conditions when TPN may be used.

    a. _____

    b. _____

    c. _____

    d. _____

    e. _____

IX. CLINICAL APPLICATIONS

1. Mr. Q's son has had a significant abdominal injury, and the trauma has disrupted his gastrointestinal system. The health care provider in charge of his case is planning to start him on total parenteral nutrition through a central venous line. Explain to Mr. Q why this is necessary for his son's nutritional well-being and what metabolic reactions can occur as a result of this therapy.

X. CASE STUDY

Mr. B., age 60, has congestive heart failure and has been receiving a diuretic as part of his therapy. When he had lab work done at the clinic, it was discovered that his potassium was low. His physician has ordered a potassium supplement for him.

1. The signs of hypokalemia include ____.
    a. nausea
    b. confusion
    c. drowsiness
    d. All of the above

2. Mr. B. is prescribed an effervescent tablet form of potassium supplement.
    a. He should place the tablet in 4 to 8 oz. of cold water or juice and wait for it to stop fizzing.
    b. The liquid should be sipped over 5 to 10 minutes.
    c. The tablet may be chewed if he does not have juice or water available.
    d. Both a and b

3. Adverse reactions that may be experienced with oral potassium supplements include all of the following except ____.
    a. depressed reflexes
    b. abdominal pain
    c. diarrhea
    d. nausea

NEW AND ALTERNATIVE DRUG THERAPIES

XII

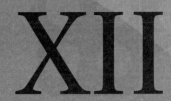

46

Complementary and Alternative Medicine

I. MATCH THE FOLLOWING

Match the term from Column A with the correct definition from Column B.

COLUMN A

_____ 1. Alternative therapies

_____ 2. Complementary and alternative medicine (CAM)

_____ 3. Complementary therapies

_____ 4. Dietary supplement

_____ 5. Efficacy

_____ 6. Fat-soluble vitamins

_____ 7. Herb

_____ 8. Herbal remedies

_____ 9. Herbal therapy

_____ 10. Minerals

_____ 11. Nutritional supplements

_____ 12. Vitamin

_____ 13. Water-soluble vitamins

COLUMN B

A. A type of complementary or alternative therapy that uses plants or herbs to treat various disorders

B. Vitamins that are generally metabolized slowly and are stored in the liver

C. Substances such as herbs, vitamins, minerals, amino acids, and other natural substances

D. Use plants or herbs to treat various disorders

E. Organic substance needed by the body in small amounts for normal growth and nutrition

F. A group of nontraditional therapies

G. Therapies such as relaxation techniques, massage, dietary supplements, healing touch, and herbal therapy used together or to "complement" traditional health care

H. Therapies used instead of conventional or Western medical therapies

I. Vitamins that are rapidly metabolized and are readily excreted in the urine

J. Substances such as herbs, vitamins, minerals, amino acids, and other natural substances

K. Effectiveness

L. Plant used in medicine or as seasoning

M. In terms of nutrition, are inorganic nutrients necessary to maintain health in the human body

II. MATCH THE FOLLOWING

Match the herb from Column A with the use from Column B.

COLUMN A

___ 1. Ginger
___ 2. Ginkgo
___ 3. Ginseng
___ 4. Kava
___ 5. St. John's wort
___ 6. Valerian
___ 7. Garlic
___ 8. Grape seed
___ 9. Chamomile
___ 10. Milk thistle
___ 11. Black cohosh
___ 12. Saw palmetto
___ 13. Echinacea
___ 14. Aloe vera
___ 15. Goldenseal

COLUMN B

A. Lowers blood sugar, cholesterol, and lipids

B. Menopause symptoms, hypercholesterolemia, and peripheral vascular disease

C. Inhibits infection and promotes healing of minor burns and wounds

D. Antiemetic, cardiotonic, antibacterial, and antitussive

E. Atherosclerosis, high blood pressure, and high cholesterol

F. Antiseptic for skin, astringent for mucous membranes, and peptic ulcers

G. Symptoms of benign prostatic hyperplasia

H. Restlessness and sleep disorders

I. Mild to moderate anxiety and as a sedative

J. Liver disease, alcoholic, and other cirrhoses

K. Raynaud disease, cerebral insufficiency, and dementias

L. Prevents and shortens symptoms and duration of upper respiratory infections

M. A tea for gastrointestinal disturbances, as a sedative, and as an anti-inflammatory agent

N. Antidepressant and antiviral

O. Enhances immune function, improves cardiovascular or CNS function

III. MULTIPLE CHOICE

Circle the letter of the best answer.

1. Herbal remedies
   a. use plants or herbs to treat various disorders.
   b. are organic substances needed by the body in small amounts for normal growth and nutrition.
   c. are vitamins that are rapidly metabolized.
   d. are vitamins that are generally metabolized slowly.

2. Complementary therapies include all of the following except
   a. relaxation techniques.
   b. massage.
   c. healing touch.
   d. surgical procedures.

3. Water-soluble vitamins
   a. are stored in the liver.
   b. are readily excreted in the urine.
   c. are dietary supplements.
   d. are usually plants used as a seasoning.

4. Vitamin E
   a. is a potent antioxidant.
   b. protects polyunsaturated fatty acids from oxidative breakdown.
   c. enhances the use of vitamin A.
   d. is found in wheat germ and rice.
   e. All of the above

5. All of the following are considered dietary supplements except _____.
   a. herbs
   b. heparin
   c. amino acids
   d. vitamins

6. Herbs are used _____.
   a. to boost the immune system
   b. to treat depression
   c. to promote relaxation
   d. All of the above

7. Echinacea should not be taken by individuals with _____.
   a. tuberculosis
   b. multiple sclerosis
   c. AIDS
   d. All of the above

8. Ginkgo biloba is used for all of the following except _____.
   a. short-term memory loss
   b. erectile dysfunction
   c. boosting stamina
   d. anxiety

9. Kava is a popular treatment for _____.
   a. reducing stress
   b. promoting sleep
   c. improving cognitive performance
   d. relieving menstrual symptoms
   e. Answers a, b, and d

10. Valerian works by _____.
    a. relaxing the muscles
    b. reducing the number of awakenings through the night
    c. preventing nerve cells in the brain from reabsorbing serotonin
    d. shortening the length of time it takes to fall asleep
    e. Answers a, b, and d

11. _____ was originally isolated from willow bark.
    a. Salicylate
    b. Coumarin
    c. Dopamine
    d. Garlic

12. Garlic is an _____.
    a. antioxidant
    b. antifungal
    c. antiviral
    d. antibiotic
    e. All of the above

13. Chamomile's uses include _____.
    a. reduce flatulence and diarrhea
    b. reduce stomach upset
    c. control motion sickness
    d. All of the above
    e. Both a and b

IV. RECALL FACTS

Indicate which of the following statements are facts with an F. If the statement is not a fact, leave the line blank.

ABOUT VITAMIN E

_____ 1. The richest sources of vitamin E are wheat germ and rice oils and the lipids of green leaves.

_____ 2. Prolonged large doses of vitamin E may result in muscle weakness, fatigue, headache, and nausea.

_____ 3. Vitamin E is not an antioxidant.

_____ 4. Vitamin E functions to enhance vitamin A use.

_____ 5. Vitamin E is capable of protecting polyunsaturated fatty acids from oxidative breakdown.

_____ 6. Vitamin E toxicity can be reversed by discontinuing the large-dose supplementation.

_____ 7. Vitamin E is a water-soluble vitamin.

ABOUT GINSENG

_____ 1. Ginseng has been called the "king of herbs".

_____ 2. Ginseng is used to improve energy and mental performance.

_____ 3. Ginseng increases the feelings of well-being.

_____ 4. Ginseng improves endurance during exercise, reducing fatigue, boosting stamina, and reaction times.

_____ 5. Ginseng is contraindicated with renal failure.

_____ 6. Ginseng should not be taken in combination with stimulants.

_____ 7. Ginseng should not be used by those taking insulin or oral antidiabetic medications without careful glucose monitoring.

V. FILL IN THE BLANKS

Fill in the blanks using words from the list below.

kava	vitamin C	minerals	toxic	relaxation techniques
blood sugar	increased sensitivity to sunlight	cholesterol	interact	sexual dysfunction
lipids	dizziness	fat-soluble	alternative therapies	massage
retinol	ultraviolet irradiation			

1. _____ are inorganic nutrients necessary to maintain health in the human body.

2. _____ is found in fresh fruit and vegetables.

3. _____ is promoted as a natural alternative to anxiety drugs.

4. Side effects of St. John's wort include _____ and _____.

5. Willow bark is purported to help with _____.

6. _____ are therapies used instead of conventional or Western medical therapies.

7. _____ vitamins are generally metabolized slowly and are stored in the liver.

8. Complementary therapies are used with traditional health care and include therapies such as _____ and _____.

9. Many botanicals have strong pharmacological activity, and some may _____ with prescription drugs or be _____ in the body.

10. Vitamin A is also called _____.

11. Vitamin D is a collective term for a group of compounds formed by the action of _____ on sterols.

12. Garlic is said to lower _____, _____, and _____.

VI. LIST

List the requested number of items.

1. List two water-soluble vitamins.

   a. _____

   b. _____

2. List five macrominerals.

   a. _____

   b. _____

   c. _____

   d. _____

   e. _____

3. List three trace minerals.

   a. _____

   b. _____

   c. _____

4. List the four fat-soluble vitamins.

   a. _____

   b. _____

   c. _____

   d. _____

5. List four herbs that affect the gastrointestinal and urinary system.

   a. _____

   b. _____

   c. _____

   d. _____

6. List three herbs that affect the cardiovascular system.

   a. _____

   b. _____

   c. _____

7. List four herbs that affect the neurologic system

   a. _____

   b. _____

   c. _____

   d. _____

8. List four types of nutritional supplements.

   a. _____

   b. _____

   c. _____

   d. _____

9. List five toxic symptoms of hypercalcemia from hypervitaminosis D.

   a. _____

   b. _____

   c. _____

   d. _____

   e. _____

VII. CLINICAL APPLICATIONS

1. You are discussing the use of nutritional supplements with a patient. List the key points that a patient should consider before he or she adds a supplement to his or her regimen.

VIII. CASE STUDY

Mr. J. has been prescribed vitamin B and C supplementation by his health care provider. You are tasked with providing information to him related to these vitamins and their use in the body.

1. You tell Mr. J. that these are water-soluble vitamins. This means that _____.
   a. they are generally metabolized slowly and are stored in the liver
   b. they are rapidly metabolized and readily excreted in the urine
   c. they are generally stored in bone tissue
   d. None of the above

2. Mr. J. asks you what foods he should eat to increase his intake of B vitamins. You tell him that eating more _____ will achieve this.
   a. meat and vegetable products
   b. seeds, especially wheat germ and rice
   c. citrus fruits
   d. Both a and b

3. You caution Mr. J. about not supplementing with extra vitamin C as megavitamin intake of vitamin C may result in _____.
   a. confusion
   b. headaches
   c. diarrhea
   d. rash